WORKING IN TEAMS

Kim Jelphs and Helen Dickinson

in association with

COMMUNITYcare

Dedication

For Ian, Karen, Paul, Gem and Zo [KJ]

First published in Great Britain in 2008 by

The Policy Press
University of Bristol
Fourth Floor
Beacon House
Queen's Road
Bristol BS8 1QU
UK

Tel +44 (0)117 331 4054
Fax +44 (0)117 331 4093
e-mail tpp-info@bristol.ac.uk
www.policypress.co.uk

North American office:
The Policy Press
c/o International Specialized Books Services (ISBS)
920 NE 58th Avenue, Suite 300
Portland, OR 97213-3786, USA
Tel +1 503 287 3093
Fax +1 503 280 8832
e-mail info@isbs.com

© Kim Jelphs and Helen Dickinson 2008
Reprinted 2010

British Library Cataloguing in Publication Data
A catalogue record for this book is available from the British Library

Library of Congress Cataloging-in-Publication Data
A catalog record for this book has been requested

ISBN 978 1 84742 033 6 paperback

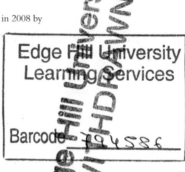

Cover design by In-text Design, Bristol
Printed and bound in Great Britain by Hobbs, Southampton

Contents

List of tables, figures and boxes

Tables

Figures

Boxes

Acknowledgements

Kim and Helen would like to acknowledge the contributions of Lynn Markiewicz of Aston Organisation Development (OD) to many of the discussions that have taken place around this book. Aston OD also allowed them to reproduce the effective partnership working inventory (Figure 4.2), the task relevancy exercise (Table 4.1), linking team and organisational objectives (Table 4.2), the role clarity review grid (Table 4.3) and the interprofessional culture review (Table 4.4). Thanks also go to Ron Church (Box 1.5), David Clutterbuck (Figure 3.3), Paul Plsek (Figure 4.4), Edward de Bono (Figure 4.5), and to everyone who allowed them to reproduce their stories and ideas.

List of abbreviations

Health and social care use a large number of abbreviations and acronyms – we note that a number of teams are starting to recognise that their use may potentially damage or obstruct communication. So, in this text we recommend that wherever possible, abbreviations should not be used, or that when used this is on the basis that all individuals understand these and interpret them in the same way. Inevitably we have had to incorporate some abbreviations. The more popular terms used in this book are set out below:

A&E	Accident and Emergency
CC	City Council
GP	General practitioner
IPE	Interprofessional education
KSA	Knowledge, skills and attributes
MBC	Metropolitan Borough Council
PCT	Primary care trust

All web references in the following text were correct at the time of printing.

Preface

Open almost any newspaper and issues of partnership working (or lack of it) leap out at you. In extreme cases it is very rare, high-profile, front-page stories – about a child death, a mental health homicide, the abuse of a person with learning difficulties or an older person dying at home alone (see Box 0.1). Here, partnership working is quite literally a matter of life and death, and a failure to collaborate can have the most serious consequences for all involved. However, most newspaper stories focusing on social issues or on public services will inevitably include reference to partnership issues – either to the need for joint working or to a social problem that is so multifaceted that an interagency response is required. Whether it be gun crime, substance misuse, prostitution, social exclusion, regeneration, third world debt, teenage pregnancy or public health, the issues at stake are often so complex that no one agency working by itself could ever hope to provide a definitive solution (or even understand the problem in its entirety).

Box 0.1: Partnership working as a matter of life or death

Following the death of Victoria Climbié in 2000, a series of reforms have taken place in children's services to promote more effective partnerships. As the then Health Secretary explained, 'there were failures at every level and by every organisation which came into contact with Victoria Climbié. Victoria needed services that worked together. Instead the [inquiry] report says there was confusion and conflict. The only sure-fire way to break down the barriers between these services is to break down these barriers altogether' (BBC, 2003).

In services for people with learning difficulties, an investigation into alleged abuse in Cornwall found that 'working relationships between the [NHS] trust and Cornwall County Council had been poor for a considerable time' and that 'social services had little involvement in the care provided by the trust, to the detriment of

---

people with learning disabilities' (Healthcare Commission/CSCI, 2006, p 7).

In mental health services, a review of mental health homicides identified a lack of partnership working as a common feature of official inquiries (and the fourth most important out of 12 contributing factors), both in health and social care, as well as with the police, housing and the independent sector (McCulloch and Parker, 2004).

In older people's services, 'thousands of people die miserable deaths alone, uncared for and in poverty, figures suggest. A study by Liberal Democrat MP Paul Burstow found around 60 people a week die alone without the support of family and friends' (BBC, 2005). In the MP's report, factors contributing to such isolation and loneliness were thought to include bereavement, illness, physical impairment, fears for personal safety, declining self-esteem, depression, retirement and a reduction in social participation, poverty and a lack of preventative health and social services (Burstow, 2005). These findings have since been re-iterated in a report commissioned by the Department of Health and Comic Relief (O'Keeffe et al, 2007), which found that, despite references to 'partnership' in a number of policy documents, abuse and neglect of older people remains prevalent in the UK.

In the health and social care trade press, interagency issues are even more prevalent (see Box 0.2 for examples). For health and social care practitioners, if you are to make a positive and practical difference to service users and patients most of the issues you face will involve working with other professions and other organisations. For public service managers, partnership working is likely to occupy an increasing amount of your time and your budget, and arguably requires different skills and approaches to those prioritised in traditional single agency training and development courses. For social policy students and policy makers, many of the issues you study and/or try to resolve inevitably involve multiple professions and multiple organisations – in both health and social care, and in the public, private and voluntary sectors. Put simply, people do not live their lives according to the categories we create in our welfare services (and in subsequent professional training and organisational structures) – real-life problems are nearly always messier, more complex, harder to define and more difficult to resolve than this.

Box 0.2: Partnership working in everyday health and social care practice

At the time of writing, the latest edition of *Community Care* magazine contained news items, opinion pieces and features about:

- child poverty and well-being
- a child death and allegations of insufficient interagency communication
- poor integration of services for children and/or young people
- the experience of people with learning difficulties in the criminal justice system
- services for children whose parents have a substance misuse problem.

Nursing Times contained pieces on:

- the link between mental health and substance misuse
- the education of nurses working in nursing homes
- the physical health of people with mental health problems
- joint working between the National Health Service (NHS) and the private sector to improve access to healthcare
- new ways of working to provide surgery and diagnostics in community settings.

In addition, *The Guardian* contained stories about:

- the link between substance misuse and crime
- gun crime in inner-city areas
- policies to tackle traffic congestion in busy cities
- the potential privatisation of the probation service
- parental mental health and the impact on children.

Policy context

In response, national and local policy increasingly calls for enhanced and more effective partnership working as a potential solution. While such calls for more joint working can be inconsistent, grudgingly made and/or overly aspirational, the fact remains that collaboration between different professions and different organisations is increasingly seen as the norm (rather than as an exception to the rule). With most new funding and most new policy initiatives, there is usually a requirement that local agencies work together to bid for new resources or to deliver the required service, and various Acts of Parliament place statutory duties of partnership on a range of public bodies. As an example of the growing importance of partnership working, the word 'partnership' was recorded 6,197 times in 1999 in official parliamentary records, compared to just 38 times in 1989 (Jupp, 2000, p 7). When we repeated this exercise for the publication of this book series, we found that there were 17,912 parliamentary references to 'partnership' in 2006 alone (although this falls to 11,319 when you remove references to legislation on civil partnerships that was being debated at the time) (for further details see www.publications.parliament.uk/pa/cm/cmhansrd.htm).

In 1998, the Department of Health issued a consultation document on future relationships between health and social care. Entitled *Partnership in action*, the document proposed various ways of promoting more effective partnerships, basing these on a scathing but extremely accurate critique of single agency ways of working (DH, 1998, p 3):

> All too often when people have complex needs spanning both health and social care good quality services are sacrificed for sterile arguments about boundaries. When this happens people, often the most vulnerable in our society ... and those who care for them find themselves in the no man's land between health and social services. This is not what people want or need. It places the needs of the organisation above the needs of the people they are there to serve. It is poor

organisation, poor practice, poor use of taxpayers' money
– it is unacceptable.

Whatever you might think about subsequent policy and practice, the fact that a government document sets out such a strongly worded statement of its beliefs and guiding principles is extremely important. In fact, there is often reason to question whether current commitments to the principle of partnership working are really as benign and well meaning as this quote implies. Like any significant change in policy emphasis and focus, the current trend towards closer joint working is probably the result of multiple interrelated factors (and many of these are explored throughout this current book series). However, the fact remains that partnership working is no longer an option (if it ever was), but a core part of all public services and all public service professions.

Aim and ethos of the 'Better partnership working' series

Against this background, this book (and the overall series of which it is part) aims to provide an introduction to partnership working via a series of accessible 'how to' books (see Box 0.3). Designed to be short and easy to use, they are nevertheless evidence-based and theoretically robust. A key aim is to provide *rigour and relevance* via books that:

- offer some practical support to those working with other agencies and professions and provide some helpful frameworks with which to make sense of the complexity that partnership working entails;
- summarise current policy and research in a detailed but accessible manner;
- provide practical but also evidence-based recommendations for policy and practice.

Box 0.3: The series at a glance

- *Partnership working in health and social care* (Jon Glasby and Helen Dickinson)
- *Managing and leading in inter-agency settings* (Edward Peck and Helen Dickinson)
- *Interprofessional education and training* (John Carpenter and Helen Dickinson)
- *Working in teams* (Kim Jelphs and Helen Dickinson)
- *Evaluating outcomes in health and social care* (Helen Dickinson)

While each book is cross-referenced with others in the series, each is designed to act as a standalone text with all you need to know as a student, a practitioner, a manager or a policy maker to make sense of the difficulties inherent in partnership working. In particular, the series aims to provide some practical examples to illustrate the more theoretical knowledge of social policy students, and some theoretical material to help make sense of the practical experiences and frustrations of frontline workers and managers.

Although there is a substantial and growing literature on partnership working (see, for example, Hudson, 2000; Payne, 2000; Rummery and Glendinning, 2000; Balloch and Taylor, 2001; 6 et al, 2002; Glendinning et al, 2002; Sullivan and Skelcher, 2002; Barrett et al, 2005), most current books are either broad edited collections, very theoretical books inaccessible for students and practitioners, or texts focusing on partnership working for specific user groups. Where more practical, accessible and general texts exist, these typically lack any real depth or evidence base – in many ways little more than partnership 'cookbooks' that give you apparently simple instructions that are meant to lead to the perfect and desired outcome. In practice, anyone who has studied or worked in health and social care knows that partnership working can be both frustrating and messy – even if you follow the so-called 'rules', then the end result is often hard to predict, ambiguous and likely to provoke different reactions from different agencies and professions. In contrast, this book series seeks to offer a more 'warts and all' approach to the topic, acknowledging the practice realities that practitioners, managers and policy makers face in the real world.

Wherever possible the series focuses on key concepts, themes and frameworks rather than on the specifics of current policy and current organisational structures (which inevitably change frequently). As a result the series will hopefully be of use to readers in all four countries of the UK. That said, where structures and key policies have to be mentioned, they will typically be those in place in England. While the focus of the series is on public sector health and social care, it is important to note from the outset that current policy and practice also emphasises a range of additional partnerships and relationships, including:

- broader partnerships (for example with services such as transport and leisure in adult services and with education and youth justice in children's services);
- collaboration not just between services, but also between professionals and people who use services;
- relationships between the public, private and voluntary sectors.

As a result, many of the frameworks and concepts in each book (although summarised here in a public sector health and social care context) will also be relevant to a broader range of practitioners, students, services and service users.

Ultimately, the current emphasis on partnership working means that everything about public services – their organisation and culture, professional education and training, inspection and quality assurance – will have to change. Against this background, we hope that this series of books is a contribution, however small, to these changes.

Jon Glasby and Helen Dickinson, Series Editors
Health Services Management Centre, School of Public Policy,
University of Birmingham

1

What is teamworking and why does it matter?

Local health and social care communities are presently facing a raft of challenges, from the need to become more dynamic and diverse while simultaneously facing pressures to become more effective and efficient to repeated restructurings, and are increasingly required to work in new ways across networks and boundaries. Effective teamworking has been seen as a potential solution to all these difficulties and more. One particular area where teamworking appears to hold much potential, however, is where health and social care communities are confronted by complex, cross-cutting issues, but are still constrained by the structural, procedural and cultural barriers which are associated with a welfare system largely designed along functional organisational lines. In other words, it has been suggested that a number of the difficulties which health and social care organisations are forced to face when trying to work together are, to some extent, a product of the design of these systems. More effective teamworking is seen as one of the potential ways in which we might overcome these problems and provide more seamless services.

The first book in this series (*Partnership working in health and social care* by Jon Glasby and Helen Dickinson) introduces the concept of partnership working and illustrates why this phenomenon has come to gain such an important place within contemporary health and social care communities. In this book we argue that, although the term 'partnership' covers a broad range of different ways of working, it is still widely used as it infers some underlying concept or principle which seems important or worth striving for. This book also demonstrates that it is not easy to make partnerships work. Although there are a range of frameworks and models available to aid partnership working, in practice it is the human factor – the individuals and groups composing the partnership – who will make it a success (or not). It is this 'people factor' in which this teamworking text is primarily interested.

This book builds on a range of theories, models and research to demonstrate the benefits (and pitfalls) inherent in teamworking, and provides frameworks and practical advice on how interagency teams may be made to function more effectively. Although teams are viewed as important organisational building blocks across a range of sectors, effective teams cannot be formed by simply grouping individuals together, even though this is often what happens in practice in health and social care. While 'partnership' has become a buzzword like 'community' or 'empowerment' in the 1980s, 'teams' and 'teamworking' have similarly become buzzwords within the fields of management and organisational behaviour in recent years. Consequently, Wildblood (2007) suggests that teams have become the (unspoken) core building blocks of many of the so-called 'fads' of modern management (for example, empowerment, business process re-engineering, quality services and management and the learning organisation). However, just because something is called a team it does not mean that the predicted benefits will simply automatically flow from this arrangement or, indeed, that teamworking is the best way to bring about particular changes. In order to gain the full range of benefits which are associated with teamworking, relationships must be forged between team members, and between teams and the wider organisational environment. Research evidence shows a range of ways in which this process might be enhanced, and this is further explored in the following chapters, as well as offering lessons about what might hinder it. A number of the mechanisms for more effective teamworking will likely be recognisable and seem, to some extent, intuitive to many of us. However, within the busy day-to-day world of service delivery, it is these basic building blocks which are often overlooked.

Despite criticisms that teamworking might be somewhat of a current fad, there is considerable evidence that effective teamworking can create a significant impact on organisational performance (see Chapter 2 for further discussion). However, it is not just the potential for improvement which is driving this agenda – there are very practical ramifications when teamworking goes wrong. Two recent high profile incidents are presented in Box 1.1 and illustrate the very real impact that can be felt by individuals and their families when teamworking and interagency teamworking is not effective.

Box 1.1: When teamworking goes wrong

One example of the implications of ineffective teamworking which has gained a great deal of media attention recently is the shooting of Jean Charles de Menezes. The young Brazilian was shot dead on 22 July 2005 while boarding a London tube train by police officers who believed that he was one of four terrorists on the run after failed suicide attacks in London the day before. The Independent Police Complaints Commission's investigation into this case highlighted a series of 'catastrophic' failures which led to the death of this innocent individual. However, the primary error appears to have been a chronic communication breakdown, both in terms of team members having clarity over what was meant by particular terms and operational processes, but also because the New Scotland Yard operations room was too noisy and chaotic for officers to be able to accurately assess information coming from surveillance officers outside Mr de Menezes' block of flats. Clearly, neither issue was insurmountable and could have potentially been avoided. The impact in this case was catastrophic for Jean Charles and very significant for the family of Jean Charles, but could have been much wider if he had, in fact, been one of the terrorist suspects.

This case was an example of where the failings of a team produced serious and negative impacts that could have been even more widespread within a different context. Although it was quite a large team, essentially it was operating within the boundaries of one organisation.

Situations become even more complex where teams are working across organisational boundaries, as happened following

---

the Indian Ocean tsunami on Boxing Day 2004. This catastrophe killed nearly 225,000 people – most were killed immediately – but in the aftermath the lives of many more individuals were affected. It is estimated that somewhere between 300 and 400 charities and non-governmental organisations operated on the ground following this disaster. The scale of funding which was committed following this event was unprecedented and to some degree is responsible for this number of agencies being mobilised to the area. However, this encouraged rivalries in spending these budgets and did not encourage collaboration. The *World disasters report* (Walter, 2005) cites the failure of aid agencies to share information as a significant reason why some people may have been disaffected with the overall response to this disaster. On the ground, a failure to share information led to a significant lack of coordination. The report calls for agencies to focus less on gathering information for their own needs and more on exchanging information with the people they seek to support. In other words, without clearly focusing on the overall task (effectively the service users), teamworking risks becoming ineffective as teams focus on their individual ends, which are not necessarily compatible with their partners.

Against this background, this chapter considers a range of definitions and distinctions which are important to understand when thinking through the different types of teamworking mechanisms which might be necessary within partnership contexts. Although teamworking in partnership settings often involves a much wider range of professional groups with different values, procedures and approaches than more traditional situations, there are certainly lessons from wider, more developed literatures which can inform these processes. The discussion suggests some of the potential benefits of teamworking, including some practical case studies of health and social communities that have developed effective teams. Finally, the chapter summarises the current policy context, highlighting how the issue of teamworking has risen to prominence within the current health and social arena, and some of the potential implications of this process.

Is teamworking in partnership settings really that different?

Although the team concept may seem by some to be overused, it is so widely applied precisely because it refers to something significant and which promises so much. Yet the creation of effective teams within partnership settings is perceived to be all the more complex. As the Audit Commission (1992, p 20) describes:

> Separate lines of control, different payment systems leading to suspicion over motives, diverse objectives, professional barriers and perceived inequalities in status, all play a part in limiting the potential of multiprofessional, multiagency teamwork. These undercurrents often lead to a rigidity within teams with members adhering to narrow definitions of their role preventing the creation of flexible responses required to meet the variety of human need presented ... for those working under such circumstances efficient teamwork remains elusive.

However, there is an important point that needs to be made here which influences both how we think about teams within the context of this book, and the types of literature which we have drawn on and incorporated. Although many partnership settings do face a number of the challenges outlined by the Audit Commission, we would question whether the various factors outlined above are specific to interagency partnership settings. Although these arenas do present major difficulties in a number of ways, 'traditionally' structured settings are also often beset by some – if not all – of these challenges. For example, hospitals might be characterised as presenting a number of these factors, but with the exception of particular functions, hospitals tend not to be thought of as partnership settings. As with many things in life this is both a blessing and a curse. In one sense this is potentially positive as there is a wide literature from which we may draw lessons when thinking about how to produce more effective teamwork in partnership settings. However, this wide literature is also problematic. There are endless texts on teams and teamworking which have originated from a variety of sources. Within the specific context of this book, there is much more literature which refers to teamworking within healthcare settings, as opposed to social care. We have tried to select the most appropriate lessons for partnerships, but inevitably there are trade-offs in terms of what has been included and what we have had to omit. Wherever possible we have tried to signpost other useful sources which students and practitioners will be able to pursue further.

Definitions and distinctions

The terms 'team' and 'teamworking' will no doubt be familiar to most of us. Indeed, it is likely that all of us have come into contact with at least one team today, whether through reading a newspaper article about a football team or the latest initiative from the Treasury team (which, incidentally was put together by a news team). Teams are ubiquitous in modern life and we refer to any number of entities as teams. Indeed, this might be part of the problem with the team concept. As outlined earlier, some commentators have suggested that team and teamworking have recently become buzzwords, and this may in part result from the fact that teams are familiar to all of us. A consequence of this is that when we talk about teams it is important that we define precisely what it is we are referring to.

Although teams are a relatively modern phenomenon, there is a long and established tradition of research into groups which is both diverse and has multiple roots. A number of disciplines have literatures relating to group working and, more recently, teams and teamwork have become central to a wide range of organisational settings and fields of research. Today it is generally acknowledged that teams and groups are different entities (although this may only be a degree of difference, rather than a fundamental divergence). Size is sometimes used as a differentiator here. Mueller et al (2000) suggest that a team is composed of between three and 15 members, while Belbin (2000) states that the maximum size for a team is no more than six to eight members. As a general rule, groups tend to be larger in size than teams, although this is by no means definitive (and we pick this point up further in Chapter 2, when we consider what research evidence suggests in terms of the link between team size and effectiveness).

The precise definition of 'team' might seem like an academic point and to some degree it is, but it has real implications in practice (see Box 1.2 for some definitions of team and aspects of teamworking that can be found within the literature). Teams differ depending on their structures, purpose, tasks, settings and team members. What is considered a team within a hospital is likely to differ to that in a primary care, mental health or respite care setting. Whether teams are temporary or permanent, where their members are from, whether membership is voluntary, what tasks the team is supposed to achieve and the level of specialised skills the team requires – all are important markers of distinction between teams. As Salas and colleagues (2000, p 343) note, 'all teams are not equal', and Appelbaum and Batt (1994) suggest that the failure to differentiate between different forms of teamworking (see Box 1.3) is partly why research has found the effects of teamworking to be inconsistent. Just as it is important for researchers to make sure that they are comparing the same things when talking about teams, a key issue for students and frontline workers when using the terms 'team' and 'teamworking' is to check out that all partners understand the same thing by these terms. As noted earlier, teams and teamworking have become buzzwords (just as partnership working has), and without being specific about what we actually mean by these terms there is a risk that their widespread use will fuel cynicism about these concepts and frontline practitioners will be reluctant to engage with these agendas. Yet, as this text argues, *real* teams are important in the delivery of quality health and social care.

Box 1.2: Helpful definitions

The Oxford English Dictionary defines teams as 'Beasts of burden yoked together' (quoted in Pearson and Jones, 1994, p 1387).

Drawing on a large review of the commercial sector literature, Cohen and Bailey (1997, p 241) describe a team as 'a collection of individuals who are interdependent in their tasks, who share responsibility for outcomes, who see themselves and who are seen by others as an intact social entity embedded in one or more larger social systems (for example, business unit or the corporation) and who manage their relationship across organisational boundaries'.

A rather more extensive definition of a team, which is quite commonly used in the literature, comes from Mohrman et al (1995, p 4), who define a team as 'A group of individuals who work together to produce products or deliver services for which they are held mutually accountable. Team members share goals and are mutually held accountable for meeting them, they are interdependent in their accomplishment, and they affect the results through interactions with one another. Because the team is held collectively accountable, the work of integrating with one another is included among the responsibilities of each member'.

West and colleagues (1998) suggest three criteria for a group to be considered a team: the group needs to have a defined organisational function and identity; the group must possess shared objectives or goals; and the team members must have interdependent roles.

The key issues and principles which we can draw from definitions of teams and groups, and which are useful to bear in mind when reading this text, suggest that:

- It is significant that there is a *shared vision* between members and that they *share objectives and goals* which are small in number, manageable and engaging.

- Moreover, in achieving these objectives there must be some element of *interdependence*, that is, the members need to work together to achieve these aims. Clegg (2005) notes that a group might have common goals, but they do not necessarily have any shared responsibility and achieving the goals is less dependent on the members working together.
- Teams tend to be *smaller in size* than groups.
- Team members tend to have *skills that are complementary* to each other in working towards achieving their goals, and members have knowledge of each other's skills.
- There is some suggestion that the team should be identifiable in a social sense – that the team is a *recognisable entity* to both those within and outside the team.
- *Not all teams are equal* – teams take different forms and it is important to bear in mind their composition and characteristics, particularly when comparing teams to one another.
- *Teams are not islands*, they are usually situated within wider social systems and interact with different teams and organisations.
- Teams need *leaders* – although these leaders may not always be single individuals who occupy positions of formal power. However, in setting a shared vision and maintaining a set of common goals some sort of leadership is generally required.

This book aims to reflect on these key issues and principles throughout, providing real-life examples and suggesting ways and means in which the difficulties and complexities of teamworking may be overcome.

McIntyre and Salas (1995) rather simplistically describe teamwork and teamworking as what a team does when it behaves as a team. In other words, teamworking is effectively a team in action. However, language is important here and can potentially impact on the way in which we think about teams. There is a tendency to think of teams as internal units (that is, not linked into wider systems), which according to McIntyre and Salas' description would mean that teamworking is simply an expression of those internal processes. However, as the example of the tsunami relief effort in Box 1.1 illustrates, teamworking often involves the collaboration of teams, as well as simply individuals.

–

One metaphor which usefully describes the way teams have tended to operate in health and social care is as castles, surrounded by a moat. Teams tend to be created and viewed as independent units, and where these prove successful there is a risk that they are left to operate alone fairly autonomously. In terms of our metaphor, the castle may have its doors open and the drawbridge lowered, but members may not actually seek to enter or leave its confines. Conversely, when times are difficult there is a tendency for teams to pull up their drawbridge and concentrate solely on internal issues. Yet, in order for the whole system to operate effectively, teams must interact with each other and the wider environment. Teams must increasingly try to lower their drawbridges and operate beyond the confines of the 'castle'; they cannot operate autonomously from the rest of the system.

Teamworking, then, to some extent, is about a manifestation of teams working together, but importantly it is also about how teams relate to wider systems. The danger of teams operating in isolation is soberly highlighted by what is called the *Nut Island effect* (Levy, 2001). In this case a committed, initially well-performing team were able to hide problems from the organisation which eventually led to a major disaster in a sewage treatment plant. The organisation gave a high degree of independence to the team as it had previously performed well, but this lack of wider linkages may have ultimately contributed to the failure of this team, which had much wider implications than for the team alone.

So far we have provided an overview of the different definitions which tend to be associated with teams and teamworking and suggested that when using these terms all partners should make sure that they understand the same things. One way of doing this within a partnership setting is by using a descriptor which outlines the range of professionals the team is composed of and the degree of collaboration between the members (Box 1.3 illustrates some of these terms). There are important distinctions between many of these terms, but they are often used interchangeably within the literature. Miller and colleagues (2001) note that notions of multidisciplinary or multiprofessional teams should not be confused with a group of professionals who work independently, but happen to liaise with one another over a period of time. There are specific criteria which teams must meet to be considered so and we need to be careful about how we demarcate teams in practice. If teams are mis-named this can potentially have a significant impact; confusion over terms may mean that team members become unclear as to the nature of the team, as may supporting organisations. This terminology matters as we expect different things from different kinds of teams and they require different forms of support.

Box 1.3: Different types of teams and groups and means of collaboration

There are a range of different types of teams which may be found within health and social care organisations. This box provides an overview of the more common, but is by no means exhaustive.

Sundstrom (1999) identified six types of teams, distinguished by the type of work they do: production; service; management; project; action/performing; and parallel teams. These teams also differ in terms of at least four further factors: level of authority within the wider organisation; time until the team is disbanded; degree of specialisation, independence and autonomy in relation to other teams; and degree to which they are interdependent within the team as well as with forces outside the team.

Teams may also be defined by their location. *Virtual teams* (or geographically dispersed teams) are a group of individuals who work across time, space and organisational boundaries, often utilising information technology (IT) to strengthen links. These are becoming an increasingly important feature of many contemporary organisations.

Self-directed or *self-managed teams* have full responsibility for the product or service which they produce, including the management of that process. The point of difference between these two types is that self-directed teams identify the goal which they are aiming to achieve.

The lean improvement methodology has recently gained much interest within the NHS (for example, Young et al, 2004; Mathieson, 2006). *Lean teams* are designed around particular processes and have complete responsibility for identifying problems, creating solutions and implementing actions to make processes as efficient and effective as possible.

In terms of health and social care partnerships, frequently used terms include:

- *Multiprofessional:* practitioners who share the same professional background who practice within two or more different specialities or branches working side by side.

- *Multidisciplinary:* practitioners from two or more different disciplines working side by side.

- *Multiagency:* practitioners from two or more different agencies working side by side. *Note:* The 'multi-' prefix implies that members of that group are not necessarily collaborating and might simply be working side by side, in parallel or sequentially towards a common problem. However, when the term 'team' is used as a suffix, it should imply that members are collaborating and working towards shared objectives.

- *Interprofessional:* practitioners who share the same professional background and practice within two or more different specialities or branches working together.

- *Interdisciplinary:* practitioners from two or more different disciplines working together.

- *Interagency:* practitioners from two or more different agencies working together. *Note:* The 'inter-' prefix denotes that there are definite interactions between the members and there is active joint collaboration towards a problem, although members may not be approaching it from the same conceptual frameworks. The 'inter-' prefix further tends to denote a greater propensity for team members to be willing to work across boundaries, which multiprofessional teams may be less willing to do. Again, whether the suffix 'team' or 'working' is used should indicate whether this collaboration is towards a specific end the members are jointly accountable for achieving.

- *Transdisciplinary teams:* members transcend their separate, conceptual and methodological orientations to overcome the disciplinary bounds that are present in multidisciplinary and interdisciplinary teams. Some commentators suggest that this is the only way to produce a truly integrated response to issues, although others have highlighted the dangers that might result from working in this way (this is considered further in Chapter 2).

Why does teamworking matter?

Teams have greater reach than individuals alone and in the complex world of health and social care no one individual has all the skills to fulfil all roles in the way a team should. Moreover, as suggested earlier in this chapter, teamworking has been seen as a potential solution to a number of structural difficulties and complexities which organisations from a range of different sectors are currently facing. As organisations have become larger and more complex in structural terms, it has become ever more important that people can work together in coordinated ways to achieve the overarching aims of their organisation. Organisations are now increasingly required to build in flexibility and to be more agile in order to be successful, and teamworking is seen as the most effective way of achieving this (Macy and Izumi, 1993; Appelbaum and Batt, 1994).

For most organisations implementing teamworking, the principle motivation is a belief that it will enhance their organisation's performance (Parker and Bradley, 2000), and a number of studies have examined the link between teamworking and performance (see

—

Chapter 2 for further discussion). In terms of health and social care, there is also some evidence that teams who work together produce better outcomes for service users, staff members and the organisation (for example, Borrill et al, 2001; Mickan and Rodger, 2005). Box 1.4 presents some of the positive impacts that teamwork is thought to be able to achieve and this makes teamworking seem a very attractive prospect. However, we must be cautious and not rush headlong into thinking that teamworking is the solution to everything (and there are clearly parallels here with the concept of partnership working itself): teams take many different forms and will not necessarily deliver all (or any) of these suggested impacts. It is important that we unravel the causal chains involved in these processes so we can be more clear about what sorts of teams are able to bring about what sorts of effects and within which contexts.

Box 1.4: Why work in teams?

Mohrman et al (1995) set out a number of reasons why organisations might implement teamworking:

- Because of the need for consistency between organisational environment, strategy and design, teams are the best way to enact the strategy of organisations.
- Teams enable organisations to speedily develop and deliver services cost effectively, while retaining high quality.
- Teams enable organisations to learn (and retain learning) more effectively.
- Cross-functional teams promote improved quality of services.
- Cross-functional teams can undertake effective process re-engineering.
- Time is saved if activities, formerly performed sequentially by individuals, can be performed concurrently by people working in teams.
- Innovation is promoted within team-based organisations because of cross-fertilisation of ideas.

- Flat organisations can be monitored, coordinated and directed more effectively if the functional unit is the team rather than the individual.
- As organisations have grown more complex, so too have their information processing requirements; teams can integrate and link in ways individuals cannot.

Cohen and Bailey (1997, p 243) suggest three major dimensions of effectiveness that result from teamworking: performance effectiveness assessed in terms of quantity and quality of outputs (in health and social care partnerships this is likely to relate to service user outcomes and satisfaction, quality of care and safety); member attitudes; and behavioural outcomes. These different levels are interesting as Parker and Bradley (2000, p 24) note that employee satisfaction has been demonstrated to link to organisational performance and those companies with high employee satisfaction have been shown to demonstrate better financial performance. Unhappy employees are more likely to be stressed, be absent from work and less likely to continue to work for a company.

Teamwork, therefore, might not only be beneficial in terms of a direct link to organisational performance, but could also create more satisfied staff members, who are more productive, less likely to be absent and more likely to enhance organisational performance. In this way, effective teamworking is thought to be able to trigger a kind of virtuous chain of events, where feedback enhances both individual and organisational performances (see Figure 1.1). Similarly, however, the converse is also thought to be true; ineffective teamworking might lead to lower staff satisfaction, negative behaviours and an inability to attract new quality staff members which might impact negatively on organisational performance, which subsequently feeds back into team morale. There is another factor which is missing from Figure 1.1, which will become increasingly important for providers and commissioners of services alike. If teamworking is effective within provider services this could potentially increase a commissioning organisation's confidence in that service and increase the possibility of that team being re-commissioned

Figure 1.1: Effective teamworking and feedback processes

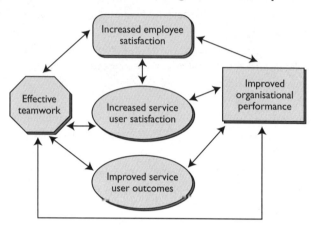

for present or extended service or being awarded more autonomy. In a policy context where the issue of 'world class commissioning' is gaining in political salience, there is more than ever a focus on the need to commission quality services effectively and safely. Therefore, commissioners will need to have an increasing interest in how care is delivered, and a key commissioner question in the future may relate to the degree to which organisations support teamworking.

Box 1.5 illustrates an example of an effective health and social care team and the impacts which this produced. Essentially this illustrates a number of the effects suggested in Figure 1.1 in practice.

Box 1.5: Example of team effectiveness

Six managers from Staffordshire County Council (CC), Birmingham CC, Dudley Metropolitan Borough Council (MBC), Walsall MBC, Sandwell MBC and Worcestershire CC have been working together to improve standards and approval panel processes for adult placement carers. The service is the adult version of fostering and offers a wide range of services, including supporting older people and facilitating respite services and long-term placements.

One of the managers commented that "by adopting a can-do attitude and working together to share problems and to support each other we have identified tangible benefits and developed a consistency of service across a wide area which we are proud of". All six local authorities have improved their standards of recruitment practices and the positive outcomes impact on service users, the managers and other staff:

- all six local authorities now use similar recruitment specifications;
- the team work together to ensure that there is feedback and scrutiny to each other about approval panels;
- more training is offered by pooling resources and working together;
- service users are now involved in the panels;
- the effectiveness and standard of care has increased;
- team members feel more supported.

Source: Provided by Ron Church (adult placement team manager)

Given the range of potential positive impacts teamworking is thought to be able to produce, health and social care workers are continually exhorted to work together to develop multidisciplinary teams and integrate services. Yet, the degree to which these positives are empirically demonstrated is to some degree questionable (and is explored further in Chapters 2 and 3). Allen and Hecht (2004) suggest that a group of individuals working together under the title of a team do not necessarily achieve more than could be achieved by a group of competent individuals working alone and that evidence shows that it is the psychological benefits or the 'romance of teams' that makes people think that their team is performing better. Furthermore, as previously demonstrated, not all teams are equal and these potential benefits should be treated with healthy scepticism. Simply describing a group of individuals as a team will not guarantee that the benefits outlined in Figure 1.2 and Box 1.5 will automatically be experienced.

Care must be taken to ensure that appropriate structures, procedures, development and training opportunities are in place in order to get the most from teams. Chapters 2 and 3 present a range of lessons from research (from both health and social care partnerships and wider relevant literatures) which suggest how effective teams may be formed and sustained. However, before this, the following section briefly considers the health and social care policy context to determine how the present onus on teamworking has developed over time.

Policy context

One of the ironies of the health and social care arena over the past quarter of a century has been that just as the concept of the 'whole patient' was being (re)-discovered through more modern perspectives of public health (acknowledging economic and socio-cultural determinants of health; for further discussion see Baggott, 2000), the professions of health and social care have become ever more specialised and narrowly focused. Since the turn of the last century, generalist workers have been progressively replaced by a diverse range of occupations and specialists who are focused on particular fields of work, problem areas, processes or client groups. With rapidly advancing knowledge and changing technologies, professionals have become ever more specialised into specific areas (although in primary care recent efforts have been made to acknowledge and value the role of the generalist; see, for example, DH, 2002a).

In practice this shift can be perceived as positive – professionals have a much more detailed understanding of a certain problem or issue – but this can prove problematic in that it is unlikely that a single person can have exhaustive knowledge of their entire profession (or, indeed other professions). Increased professional specialisation has led to the internal fragmentation of health and social care organisations, requiring professionals to work more closely and with a wider range of colleagues internally within their organisations. Over this period there has also been a growing recognition that individuals often have multifactoral problems, which a single agency alone cannot solve and which requires the input of multiple agencies. That is, while agencies are becoming increasingly internally specialised, requiring professional groups to work together, they are also being called on to work with outside agencies to provide services around the needs of individuals. Consequently, no one professional is likely to be able to provide all the support and assistance that an individual with chronic or complex needs requires, and we are starting to see expansive care pathways emerging for many conditions. Increasingly, the implication is that each profession and expert system is necessarily required to overlap with others. Teamworking has been seen as one way to work more effectively over both these internal and external boundaries.

Consequently, since the early 1970s we have started to see reference to entities such as primary care teams (BMA, 1974), community mental health teams (DH, 2002b), intermediate care teams (DH, 2000) and any other number of teams organised around specific conditions or client groups. Not only are these teams thought to simplify 'patient journeys' and move towards the more seamless delivery of care, but also to reduce duplication, cut costs and potentially increase the productivity of the system. As one NHS Management Executive (1993) report suggests:

> The best and most cost-effective outcomes for patients and clients are achieved when professionals work together, learn together, engage in clinical audit of outcomes together, and generate innovation to ensure progress in practice and service.

Indeed, *The NHS Plan* (DH, 2000) goes as far as to suggest that poor teamworking is one of the reasons why the NHS has failed to deliver on healthcare priorities in the past. This document claims that the NHS is a '1940s system operating in a 21st-century world', which failed due to its 'old-fashioned demarcations between staff and barriers between services' (DH, 2000, p 10). Under this reading it is thought that somehow working in teams can compensate for the limitations of current organisational structures, and reduce the irritations that these cause within the everyday work of staff members. However, it remains to be seen to what degree this has actually become a reality

—

in health and social care. Aims and objectives for teams often remain more rhetoric than reality; in practice effective teamworking often remains more apsirational and idealised than realised.

One of the difficulties in trying to summarise the policy context in respect to teamworking is that so many different areas of policy impact on teams and teamworking. Health and social care communities have recently undergone, and are undergoing, some fairly fundamental changes in terms of their structures and configurations, all of which have had, and are having, impacts on the employment conditions and allegiances of staff members. In recent years we have seen a more pronounced split in terms of commissioners and providers of services, accompanied by diversification of provision (in both health and social care). We have seen the separation of adults and children's social care services, prison healthcare services coming under the auspices of the NHS and so on. Not only do such structural changes disrupt existing relationships between individuals and agencies, but they also fundamentally alter the compositions of traditional teams, and these have real impacts on the ways in which they are able to work together.

Yet structures are just one thing which impact on teams. The introduction of various legal flexibilities means that in some areas social care staff are transferring to health employment (or vice versa). The health and social care workforce is changing significantly with ongoing professionalisation and educational reforms, in addition to the influx of a number of overseas professionals. A whole range of policy initiatives have been launched over the past decade which have the potential to significantly affect the nature and capacity of the health and social care workforce further (for example, DH, 1999, 2000, 2002a, 2002c). Nor does it seem likely that such changes are going to stop. Days of stability for health and social care organisations seem to be a thing of the past and increasingly it will be up to individuals and teams to make sense of this context and lead through change (Martin, 2003). These changes clearly have important implications for teamworking and individuals may find themselves working with people from a wider range of sectors and backgrounds than ever before. Therefore, this text, with its subject matter of partnerships and teamworking, is very timely.

—

Reflective exercises

1. Think about the key principles of teams suggested in this chapter. To what degree are these reflected in your understanding of teamworking?

2. Ask a colleague or friend how they would define teams/teamworking. How does this compare to your understanding?

3. Make a list of teams that you have encountered recently, both in your professional and personal life. Thinking about the definitions of teams offered in this chapter, do you think these teams have the characteristics suggested?

4. Have any of the teams you thought about in response to the previous question produced any of the positive effects outlined in this chapter which teamworking is thought to be able to achieve? Were there any negative impacts?

5. Think of a team in the public eye that you believe embodies teamwork. What does it do that makes you perceive it as a real team?

Further reading and resources

Readers may find some of the websites listed below useful as they contain information on the topic of teams. They include:

- The Integrated Care Network, which aims to promote integration within policy for service improvement: www.integratedcarenetwork. gov.uk
- The knowledge exchange, which is a web-based community where health and social care managers connect to share information and exchange ideas: www.theknowledgexchange.co.uk
- The National Library for Health, which contains a wealth of information including briefings for managers on policy areas and hot topics: www.library.nhs.uk
- The Canadian Health Services research foundation site, which has an electronic DVD that discusses enhanced teamworking to improve patient care: www.chsrf.ca/research_themes/workplace_e.php

Key introductory teamworking texts include:

- Adair's (1986) *Effective team building*
- Payne's (2000) *Teamwork in multiprofessional care*
- West and Markiewicz's (2004) *Building team-based working*

2

What does research tell us?

There is no shortage of books on 'how to do teamworking' and 'how to build better teams' available from any local library or bookshop. Various claims have been made concerning the impacts that effective teamworking may have on both individuals and organisations, but similarly there are several reports where these assumed benefits have not always been fully realised. Salas et al (2000, p 340) note, 'many organisations have, in the past, assumed that a team is a mere collection of individuals and, as such, assumed that merely putting members together would result in effective performance, but this is not true'. While there are a range of potential mitigating factors which might blunt the impact of teamworking, some commentators have also questioned the degree to which these presumed benefits have been demonstrated within a health and social care context. Zwarenstein and Reeves (2000, p 1022) describe this context as replete with rhetoric about the value of teamworking, but a lack of evidence to support the notion that it is necessarily a 'good thing' – hence their conclusion 'what's so great about collaboration?'.

Against this background, this chapter reviews the claims made for teamworking and questions the extent to which these are evidence-based within health and social care settings. The chapter then goes on to consider what helps and hinders teamworking, referring to some of the hot topics and frameworks which Chapters 3 and 4 draw on. In the course of these discussions we cite practical examples from various health and social care communities to illustrate these points.

What is teamworking supposed to achieve and what does the research tell us?

In *Partnership working in health and social care* (Glasby and Dickinson, 2008) it was suggested that there is a lack of evidence demonstrating that partnership working necessarily leads to better outcomes for service users. Similarly, despite the range of benefits which have been claimed for teamworking, there is limited evidence clearly demonstrating these positive effects within health and social care research. Irvine et al (2002) note that even where members recognise their interdependence, there has only been limited success in terms of health outcomes such as length of stay, improved coordination and integration of services, or, in how well stakeholders interact. However, as with partnerships, this may in part result from the difficulties which are inherent in evaluating interagency teamworking, given different objectives for teams, variations in local contexts and cultures and the variety of different theories and methods which have been used in research. These evaluation challenges may have had more impact on the nature of the evidence base than teams and teamworking lacking impact per se. This section considers the areas where research indicates teamworking in interagency settings has demonstrated a positive impact.

Organisational performance

A range of different theorists, drawing on research from a variety of different sectors and organisations, have suggested that teamworking can lead to better performance and productivity (for example, Pasmore et al, 1982; Weldon and Weingart, 1993; Appelbaum and Batt, 1994, to name but a few). Macy and Izumi (1993) found that team development initiatives were the interventions that brought about the largest effects on the financial performance of organisations. However, as Parker and Williams (2001, p 42) observe, 'the beneficial effects are not as great or consistent as we would expect from the theory, particularly when it comes to enhancing organisational performance'. Although Borrill et al (2001) note a significant and negative relationship between the percentage of staff working in teams and the mortality rates associated with these hospitals (that is, the greater percentage of teamworking, the lower the mortality), there is little evidence from studies of health and social care partnerships which demonstrates that teamworking improves organisational performance significantly.

As suggested earlier, this may be a product of the difficulties inherent in demonstrating a link between the effectiveness of a team/teams working together and an entire organisation's performance. Moreover, as previously noted, teams are not islands. Although some individual teams may be working together effectively, this might not serve to positively impact on the wider organisation's overall performance if they are not interacting with wider teams or organisational structures.

Safety

There is a fairly well established evidence base which suggests that in the NHS more effective teamworking is associated with safer working practices. Better teamworking is thought to be underpinned by more effective communication and interaction between team members which lowers the risk of unsafe behaviours and practices (safety is discussed further in Chapter 3). The *2003 NHS staff survey* (Healthcare Commission, 2004) suggested that the greater the number of staff working in well-structured teams, the fewer errors, near-misses and injuries that tended to occur. There are also a range of accounts within the literature where poor teamworking has contributed to poor safety.

Reduced costs

Although, as suggested above, there is not unequivocal evidence demonstrating a link between interagency teamwork and organisational performance, a number of international studies have concluded that effective interagency teams have produced cost savings in the care of older patients (Kane et al, 1992; Sommers et al, 2000; Hébert et al,

2005). In these cases, savings have generally come through reduced rates of emergency hospital admissions and fewer cumulative days patients have spent either in hospital or in institutional care. As there are generally much higher costs associated with hospital and institutional settings than care provided either in individuals' own homes or daycare locations, these teams can provide a larger volume of support and at lower costs. This community-based input serves to have a preventative effect, supporting individuals in their own homes for longer.

Johri et al (2003) have suggested that it is the incentive of financial reward which comes through this downward substitution (that is, more input at primary/community level than in acute/institutional settings) that is a motivator for teams to work together effectively with the aim of maintaining individuals within their own home. However, where this reward is not kept by the team, there is less incentive for it to operate quite as effectively. This suggests that incentives can have a positive effect on teamworking, and a lack of incentive could potentially mitigate against this outcome of cost saving.

Improved service user satisfaction

Clearly, these cost savings are an incentive for the agencies involved, but maintaining individuals within community settings may also impact positively on service user satisfaction. A key strand of current government policy relates to maintaining individuals in their own homes and communities, rather than in acute or hospital-based settings, and central government argues that this is what individuals want in terms of their care (see, for example, DH, 2006). However, as Kodner and Kay Kyriacou (2000) note, this cannot be assumed to be consistent across all users receiving a service; individual preference will mean that some will inevitably be more satisfied than others with particular arrangements.

However, it is not just in terms of cost savings or where care is delivered that team working can impact on service user satisfaction. Borrill et al (2003) found links between teamworking processes, participation, support for innovation and reflexivity and patient satisfaction. The research team suggest a significant relationship between the level of support team members received from their colleagues and patient satisfaction.

Improved access

Teamworking in partnerships has also been demonstrated to impact on other aspects of service delivery. Brown et al (2003) report on an interagency team that resulted in a quicker response between referral and assessment within services for older people, and a system to which individuals found they could more easily self-refer. In this study, the locally based health and social care team with one access point (general practitioner [GP] practice) provided easier direct access to services for individuals. This study also noted a slight increase in the numbers of individuals being admitted to institutional care from the interagency team. Jones (2004) suggests that this might be the result of team members sharing more information and therefore having a fuller picture of the risks posed for individuals remaining within their own homes. Although some other studies have tended to use admission to institutional care as a sign that teamworking has not been effective (that is, that teams had not worked together effectively enough and so individuals had been admitted to secondary care settings), in this case Jones argues that the team was functioning effectively, communicating much more and as a result individuals were living in the most appropriate settings.

Within mental health services, an extensive and systematic review of community-based services found that community team-based psychiatric services led to a reduction in suicide rates, improved patient engagement and were more acceptable to service users (Tyrer et al, 1999). Similarly, community mental health teams have been shown to make specialist care more available to those with severe mental illnesses, who would not previously have received care from mental health services (Jackson et al, 1993), and provide more seamless services (Katon et al, 1999).

Impact on staff members

In an NHS study, Borrill and colleagues (2001) found that those individuals working in clearly defined secondary care teams had lower levels of stress than those not working in teams or working in loose groupings. The researchers suggest that teamworking provides more social support to individuals and role clarity than those not working within teams or who are only quasi members. Borrill et al (2001, p 162) go on to suggest that it is this social support and clarity of role which accounts for the difference in stress levels between membership types, suggesting; 'it is as though, by working in a team, team members achieve a shared level of self-sufficiency that buffers team members from the inadequacies of their organisations'.

However, there is a caveat here; these impacts were only shown to result where there were *real* interdependencies and social support between team members. The *2003 NHS staff survey* (Healthcare Commission, 2004) demonstrates that working in a 'team' actually predicts a *higher* level of staff injuries and stress. However, working in a *well-structured* team predicted lower levels of injuries and illness among staff and also *lower* levels of errors and near-misses witnessed by staff. Furthermore, Sommers et al (2000) suggest that the reduced rates of hospitalisation detected in their study came from teams where individuals were most satisfied with their working relationships – but the opposite is also true of teams who are not satisfied. Ultimately humans are driven by a need for social support. Only when individuals feel as though they really are team members would this sense of social support be expected to result. Other research also points to teamworking as a key to increasing staff commitment and satisfaction (Schultz and Schultz, 1988; Goodman and Svyantek, 1999).

Thus, teamworking is thought to have a significant effect on members, providing both social support and clarity around their role and tasks. All these aspects reduce uncertainty and stress and increase satisfaction. Where individuals fail to understand their role, this is one of the biggest causes of stress within the workplace. Box 2.1 illustrates an example of a rehabilitation team where staff members did not fully understand either their own roles or the roles of their colleagues and the implications this had. There is a wealth of research from the human resources field which suggests that the more satisfied staff members are, the less likely they are to be absent from work and the more likely they are to remain within the organisation. Organisations which have unsatisfied staff members typically have higher rates of absences and higher turnover of staff members. Therefore teamworking has been demonstrated to have the potential to have significant impacts on relationships, recruitment and retention – *under certain conditions.*

Box 2.1: Implications of teams without clarity of vision or roles

Members of a newly established multidisciplinary rehabilitation team were struggling to work together effectively. The atmosphere was poor, relationships were not well developed and people were starting to go off sick. No development time had been invested in the team and eventually the team leader asked for help. The team had a development day with a skilled facilitator and it transpired that much of the friction within the team was associated with a misunderstanding of roles and confusion over the vision and philosophy of the team.

Care assistants who had previously worked on inpatient wards were working with clients in a way that conflicted with the models of independence that the therapists within the team were trying to promote. For example, a patient had come out of a one-hour session with a physiotherapist where he had to undertake exercises to facilitate independence, but when he went into the communal area the care assistants did tasks for the individual that the physiotherapist had tried to encourage him to do himself. The care assistants thought they were helping, as this was the work they were familiar and confident with. The care assistants did not feel comfortable supervising individuals while they carried out their own tasks and were much more used to doing these things for people. Once the team could discuss their philosophy of care and how each team member could contribute to the overall vision and goals of the team, the atmosphere, relationships and quality of care improved significantly.

Team innovation

In her framework of synergy, Hastings (1996) suggests one form of synergy that partnership might produce – innovation (for further discussion see Glasby and Dickinson, 2008). Interagency teams bring together people with different perspectives and backgrounds, which should produce different and more innovative solutions to problems; single agencies acting alone may not be able to produce such solutions. Within the NHS, multiprofessional teamworking has been linked to innovation by Borrill et al (2001). The researchers note that where team processes are effective, this greatly enhances the degree to which teams are innovative.

These findings have also been corroborated by other studies (for example, Hodges and Hernandez, 1999). However, this is not necessarily reflective of all contexts. Dickinson et al (2007) provide a case study of a care trust leadership team and suggest that in setting up the organisation, too much continuity with the past was maintained to ease this change process, but at the expense of innovation. Although under some circumstances teamworking might lead to greater innovation, there are a range of potential confounding factors that might impact on this process.

Overall, therefore, it seems as though effective teamworking has the potential to impact on a number of areas of health and social care service provision, performance, staff satisfaction and outcomes for service users. However, it is important to note that the opposite is also true, that is, a failure for teams to operate effectively – or indeed as 'real' teams – might lead to stressed-out staff, poor team and organisational performance and worse outcomes for service users. Also worth noting is that these impacts are not guaranteed just because we call a group of people a team. There are certain things which need to be in place in order for teams to be effective, and there are a range of factors which hold the potential to limit possible impacts. Box 2.2 presents a patient's story of their experience receiving treatment from an integrated cancer team and the impact this had on the nature and quality of care delivered. This clearly demonstrates the impact which teamworking can have on the quality of care a patient receives (we discuss the issue of leadership further below). The remainder of this chapter gives an overview of what helps and what hinders teamworking.

Box 2.2: Patient story of receiving care from an integrated team

'I really believed that the multidisciplinary specialist team caring for me worked as a team, as they all knew what the current situation was and I never felt that they didn't know. As a patient in a very vulnerable position, I felt confident and reassured and I did not have to keep responding to the same questions from different people. This situation carried on after discharge. For example, if I saw the registrar it was as good as seeing the consultant as they shared information and decisions really well and I felt included and part of the team.

I think the consultant was a real leader as he always explained to the team what was going on and he always took people through my case. He shared information in a way that people could remember so when they saw me again they had a real understanding of the complicated issues and I am sure this was because of the way the consultant explained things ... it was his style. However, when the same team was lead by a different consultant it was a totally different experience. He talked as if I wasn't there and was dismissive if I tried to contribute. It was also obvious that the rest of the team were different – they didn't ask questions or comment at all and I didn't feel as comfortable or confident.'

Source: Personal communication

What helps and hinders teamworking?

In the previous section we outlined what the research tells us about some of the potential effects of teamworking. Yet, as this section and numerous commentators suggest, teamworking is not easy to make a reality (Ingram and Desombre, 1999; Irvine et al, 2002). There are a number of barriers which may prevent effective teams from being forged. In terms of healthcare, West and Slater (1996) estimate that less than one in four teams have built effective teamworking practices and so there is a large gap between the rhetoric of what healthcare teams could potentially achieve and what they do in practice. Anning and Edwards (1999) suggest it is often the case that professionals are simply exhorted to multiagency teamworking with little training or guidance. Indeed, in the UK, much recent policy has demanded the formation of new teams, and organisations have been measured on whether they exist, rather than necessarily whether they are working effectively. Yet, despite the volume of research dedicated to teams, there is no single prescription for an effective team. This section aims to give an overview of some of the things that help and hinder teamworking, and links to the frameworks provided in Chapter 4 which aim to aid readers in producing more effective teams in practice.

Borrill and colleagues (2001) suggest a model of team effectiveness based on relationships between team inputs, process and outputs (Figure 2.1). This model suggests various potential variables in terms of inputs and team processes which could have a significant impact on the range of outputs which might be expected to flow from teamworking. Although presented here as a linear model, in reality the various factors are likely to be much more intertwined and complex than a simple relationship. Moreover, some of these factors will be more relevant to some organisational and team contexts than others.

Structure

The range of structural barriers which exist within health and social care teams are fairly well rehearsed and are the result of the quite

Figure 2.1: Model of team effectiveness

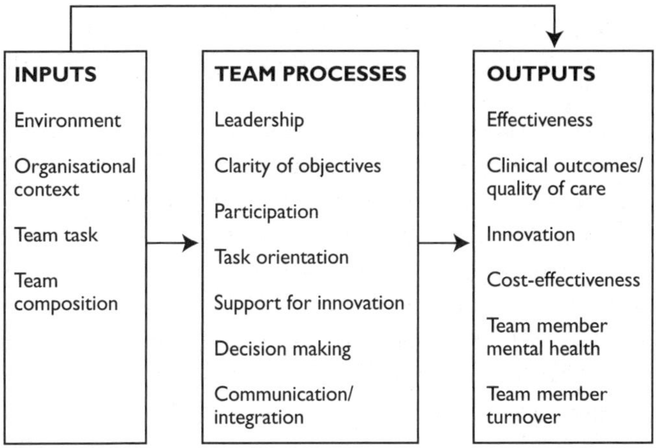

INPUTS	TEAM PROCESSES	OUTPUTS
Environment	Leadership	Effectiveness
Organisational context	Clarity of objectives	Clinical outcomes/ quality of care
Team task	Participation	Innovation
	Task orientation	
Team composition	Support for innovation	Cost-effectiveness
	Decision making	Team member mental health
	Communication/ integration	Team member turnover

Source: Adapted from Borrill et al (2001)

different ways in which these services have developed. Health and social care agencies tend to have different procedures, standards, measures of effectiveness, accountability lines, management styles (for further discussion, see Poxton, 2004), and health and social care staff members tend to have different pay rates, leave entitlements, access to funds for training and development and so on. In the UK, health and social care services have different entitlement bases (with health services being free at the point of delivery and some social care services being means-tested) and clearly this can cause barriers in health and social care staff members working together effectively. Linking in to this, there are also issues over the resourcing of these services, and some teams may find that one of the partners holds significantly more of the budget than others (conversely others may hold more of the legitimacy).

Although central government has to some extent tried to address some of these structural issues (for example, by promising to align finance and budget cycles and merge inspection authorities), it still remains the case that team members may find themselves having to contend with quite different practices, procedures and accountabilities in everyday life, although as suggested earlier, these characteristics are not necessarily restricted just to partnership settings. What this can mean in practice is confusion over accountability. While these are surmountable differences for effective teams, in practice they can take much work to overcome.

In *Partnership working in health and social care* (Glasby and Dickinson, 2008) a detailed overview was presented of the impacts of structural change on partnership working. One thing that most commentators agree on is that, although structures do to some degree present barriers to producing effective interagency teams, changing structures in themselves are insufficient to produce integrated service delivery (Burns and Pauly, 2002; van Wijngaarden et al, 2006). In an attempt to deliver care ever more organised around the needs and wishes of individuals it would be impossible to completely demolish all the structural barriers which professionals might encounter within an arena which is becoming ever more diversified. As Robinson and Cottrell (2005, p 557) describe, 'with the creation of multi-agency teams ... boundary disputes are not dispensed with. These boundary disputes shift, the points of tension re-locate from where they would be if the multi-agency teams did not exist'. The key principles which were outlined in Chapter 1 suggested that teams need to have a shared vision and joint objectives to work together, and accountability for delivering these. As such, simply structuring a group of people together and removing the barriers which might hinder them working together will be insufficient to produce an effective team. By giving teams interesting tasks which members really engage with, teams can be made more effective (Hackman, 1990).

Team composition and roles

Although a seemingly obvious and elementary point, effective teams must be composed of the right individuals with the right skills for the objectives of the team. Indeed it would seem counter-intuitive to establish a team and actively search for the wrong kinds of individuals. However, often within a health and social care environment we do not have the luxury of building teams from scratch as some other industries do. Usually it is the case that we need to shape and develop existing teams. Furthermore, over time things change. It is a worthwhile exercise to periodically review who is within a team and whether there is still the right mix of individuals for the task in hand.

Team members should have the necessary skills which complement each other in terms of what they can contribute to the team and to the overarching objectives of the team. Just as the task should engage the entire team, so too should individuals be charged with tasks which they can clearly see contribute to the overall aims of the team in a significant way (see Box 2.3 for an example). As we suggest throughout much of this book, it is the social processes which go on within teams that make individuals feel supported and secure. Therefore, for effective teamwork it is necessary for all individuals to feel that they are involved and are meaningfully contributing to the overall aims and objectives of the team. Not everyone is alike and that is a strength of both teamworking and partnerships; different perspectives and skills can be incredibly productive if harnessed effectively, but learning to work with this difference can be a difficult process. In a situation where one or two individuals become disengaged it is all too easy for this pattern to spread to other members and quickly lead to the production of an ineffective team whose interrelationships have broken down. It is also worth noting at this point that, in reality, individuals tend to belong to more than one team, although their degree of engagement with each will likely be quite different in practice.

Box 2.3: Demonstrating the importance of an individual's contribution to team activities

One of the authors was brought in to evaluate an integrated team for disabled children comprising local authority, education and healthcare staff. The team largely seemed to be functioning quite effectively, but there were a few specific issues which were highlighted as problematic. One such issue was the attitude of the staff manning the reception area. Some of the other team

—

members felt that the reception staff could be perceived as rude by families as they arrived for appointments.

The team set about an exercise trying to think through how they could improve outcomes for service users. At this point one of the reception staff asked the facilitator why they were involved in this discussion, because "this wasn't anything to do with them". The facilitator then asked the reception staff member what they did. The receptionist outlined their role, stating that they greeted families at reception, answered the telephone and informed members of the team if someone had arrived for an appointment or left a message for them. The facilitator pointed out that, in fact, the receptionist had a crucial role as they formed the first impression of the team and would effectively set the tone of the following meeting by their attitude towards people as they arrived.

Following these discussions, a marked change in the attitude of the receptionist was noted. This individual was much friendlier with families and staff members, and seemed to be much more content in their role now that they could see the way in which they made a contribution to the quality of care offered by the team.

Stevens and Campion (1994) suggest that focusing on the knowledge, skills and abilities (KSAs) of team members is a much better way of forming effective teams than simply recruiting members on the basis of their personality traits or dispositions. They argue that there are specific KSAs which are required for effective teamwork, for example:

- conflict resolution
- collaborative problem solving
- communication
- goal setting and performance management
- planning and task coordination.

Selecting individuals on the basis of these KSAs is suggested as being as, if not potentially more, important than the technical abilities of team members (and a number of these factors are covered in greater detail in Chapters 3 and 4). Stevens and Campion (1994) argue that individuals who work in teams have a wider range of technical skills because of the demands that teamwork puts on individuals in terms of flexibility and versatility. While they do not deny the importance of technical skills, they argue that the particular KSAs which are required to work well together with others are crucial in developing effective teams. Although the health and social care system invests in training for individual technical capacities (often with a poor return) it has not historically invested in people developing these types of skills and the confidence to work in teams. Additional training still tends to be valued over development in these areas, and it is often presumed that individuals will have these skills. There is perhaps much that health and social care organisations could learn from other organisations such as the armed forces and some areas of manufacturing where investment is made in developing these types of skills, and not just in developing technical abilities.

We suggested earlier in this chapter that one of the ways in which partnership working is thought to improve performance is through the innovation synergy which is formed by bringing together different perspectives to produce different solutions to problems. While a number of studies have shown that diversity of skills within a team can have a positive impact on the performance of tasks (for example, Guzzo and Dickson, 1996), bringing together a heterogeneous group of individuals also brings with it a range of potential barriers. The more diverse and different team members are from each other, the more likely it is that some individuals might have stereotypical or negative reactions towards one another. As such, it is important that certain mechanisms are put in place, such as the chance for informal communication for individuals to start to get to know each other beyond first perceptions. Diverse teams do hold the potential to be more able to deal with a range of issues due to the wider characteristics and skills set they will possess. However, in order for these to be drawn on and utilised to the best of their abilities, appropriate interrelations and communication methods must exist between team members (this point is drawn out further in the following two chapters).

—

Professional boundaries and values

The issue of whether professional boundaries should be blurred or moved and whether successful interprofessional working should involve members of teams taking on parts of the roles of others in moving towards transdisciplinary working is a key area of debate within the literature. As illustrated earlier, there are a number of well-documented structural barriers to effective teamworking, but there are further implications which flow from staff members belonging to different agencies and differing professions. Some commentators have referred to the 'tribalism' of health and social care professions (Hunter, 1996), which can potentially lead to clashes of values and beliefs (Carpenter and Barnes, 2001), or the tendency for particular professional groups to try and gain dominance over others within multiprofessional settings (Cott, 1997). Consequently, some commentators have suggested that for successful interdisciplinary teamwork, individuals need to be much more flexible and not adhere to their professional boundaries in a strict manner. It has been suggested that one potential way of making multiprofessional teams more effective would be to blur the boundaries between professions and allow all professionals to take on certain aspects of some roles. 'Interdisciplinary care, whilst not denying the importance of specific skills, seeks to blur the professional boundaries and requires trust, tolerance and a willingness to share responsibility' (Nolan, 1995, p 306).

However, other commentators have vehemently spoken out against such a move. For example, Rushmer (2005; Rushmer and Pallis, 2002) suggests that boundary blurring has the potential to significantly undermine the effectiveness of teams. This view of role blurring suggests that it might cause teamworking to break down, as individuals will be unsure of what it is their role entails and what it is they should be doing. Rushmer argues that there is a significant difference between interprofessional working and blurred boundary working. Where professionals work together interprofessionally, each knows what their role is and how they contribute to the overall aims and objectives of the team and where they will need to work with others in order to deliver certain tasks. Where boundaries are blurred this leads to confusion over who should do what, causes difficulty with role clarity, increasing stress and potentially threatens professional identity (see Box 2.4 for an example).

Box 2.4: Role clarity and boundary blurring

In a large cross-sectional study of multidisciplinary community mental health teams, Onyett et al (1997) found there were significant differences in job satisfaction and stress levels between professions. Consultant psychiatrists, social workers, nurses and psychologists were particularly stressed, but occupational therapists and psychiatrists were much more satisfied with their jobs. The research team suggest that this might be due to the social workers having more marginal positions within the team as a result of them being employed by a different agency. Conversely it could be due to a clash of the 'social' values of these workers in a medically dominated mental health context. However, they also suggested that it could be due to 'role blurring' with the healthcare workers. This blurring may have potentially led to a loss of professional identity and much less role clarity. It is this lack of role clarity combined with a marginal position that increased stress and reduced job satisfaction.

Education

Over the past 30 years there have been ever more increasing calls for the interprofessional education (IPE) of health and social care professionals. The third book in this series (*Interprofessional education and training* by John Carpenter and Helen Dickinson) considers the issue of IPE in more detail, but we give a brief overview here as it is often presented as an important factor in producing more effective teams. The premise of IPE is that by learning together, professions will understand each other better and be able to work together more effectively, providing better quality of care for patients. By learning together, professions should value aspects of each other's practice more and be able to set aside negative stereotypes (Barr et al, 2005). IPE may take place at a number of different times during professionals' careers (pre-qualifying or post-qualifying) and can take a number of different forms (implicit/explicit, particular client group/general, interactive/didactic, individual/collective and so on). Clearly, given the range of different potential approaches which IPE may contain, it might prove to have different impacts dependent on the structure and theories underpinning IPE programmes and this can make it quite difficult to generalise between programmes in practice.

Despite this, a range of evaluations have noted changes in staff members' attitudes and perceptions, knowledge and skills, behaviours, organisational practice and outcomes for service users as a result of IPE. A number of these changes are associated strongly with the shift towards more effective teamworking, particularly by overcoming some of the potential barriers referred to above. However, evaluations of IPE have been quite roundly critiqued by some academics for their robustness and it has been suggested that a number of evaluations have used unverified or inappropriate tools (Freeth et al, 2002). IPE is currently a key concern for a number of governments internationally, but as Craddock et al (2006) suggest, unless robust evaluations of the different models of IPE are produced it will remain somewhat of a fad which has the potential to fade, rather than develop as an informed practice.

Leadership

Like IPE, there is another book in this series which deals in detail with the issues of managing and leading in interagency settings. This, too, is often presented as an important factor in building effective teams and so a brief overview of the key issues is presented here. However, for those interested in the topic we would suggest reading this sister volume to complement what is inevitably a brief snapshot below (*Managing and leading in inter-agency settings*, by Edward Peck and Helen Dickinson). Leadership is probably one of the most written about topics in terms

—

of organisational studies. There are no end of texts claiming that leadership is the solution to any number of organisational problems and that leadership style impacts extensively on the performance of an organisation. However, much of this is in the form of managerial 'cookbook' literature, and relates to single organisations in the private sector, predominantly based in the US, rather than to interagency, UK public sector settings. This means that any conclusions must be considered carefully for their application within different contexts.

Leadership in a traditional sense tends to be associated with hierarchical command and control systems. Power resides with the executive, who direct those in the levels beneath, with ultimate accountability usually also residing with the top. These forms are often associated with 'great-man' styles of leadership, or with leaders who are charismatic and are easily able to influence followers. While these notions of leadership pervade the literature in a variety of forms, they are often seen as inappropriate to multiagency settings where team members might have different line managers, or modes of accountability (for an example of this debate, see Klijn and Koppenjan, 2000). It is further suggested that following a traditional model of leadership would mean that teams would not be ultimately responsible for taking decisions which are imperative to their everyday operation; the responsibility for this would likely lie elsewhere.

As a consequence, it has been increasingly suggested that distributed or shared leadership might instead produce more effective teamworking. In practice, this would mean that responsibility for decisions and leadership would be spread throughout the team, with the team sharing responsibility for maintaining its members as a social entity. More effective teams have been associated with these practices as it is suggested that this engages all team members in these acts, rather than members acting in a more passive role where they are told what to do. Such a form of leadership also requires very different styles and different ways of influencing others than 'traditional forms' would suggest.

However, it is important to note that this division between traditional and distributive leadership is not as straightforward or simple as would first appear. As already re-iterated, the concept of partnership covers a multiplicity of different working arrangements, some of which will actually be quite similar to 'traditional' settings with hierarchically derived authority and rules. The issue of leadership is actually more nuanced than much of the literature suggests and leaders would be well served by paying close attention to the context(s) in which they are operating and the resources available to them, not only in terms of authority relationships, but also personal linkages, the predominant sense-making mechanisms within the organisations and the ways in which they 'perform' leadership.

Figure 2.2 outlines Kogler Hill's (2004) model of leadership which illustrates the many different roles team leaders tend to be required to fulfil. As this model helpfully highlights, the nature, function and level of interventions that leaders are required to make will depend on what kind of activities leaders need to perform, with whom and

Figure 2.2: Kogler Hill's (2004) model of leadership

Factors which mediate leaders' decisions:
- Type of intervention
- Level of intervention
- Function of intervention

Internal team

External team

Task

Relational

Environmental

Task	Relational	Environmental
Clarify goals	Coaching	Networking
Establish structure	Collaborating	Advocating
Decision making	Managing conflict	Negotiating support
Training	Building commitment	Buffering
Standard setting	Satisfying needs	Assessing
	Modelling principles	Sharing information

Team effectiveness
Performance/development/maintenance

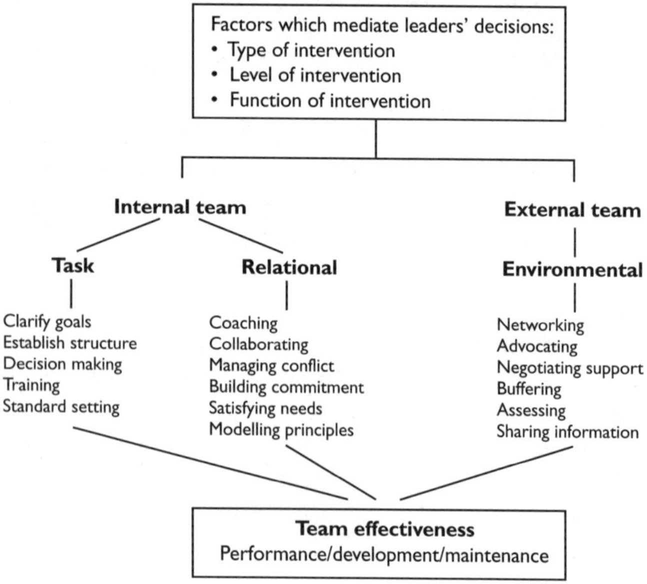

where. An example of the use of this model is outlined in Box 2.5 and demonstrates the implications of this model in practice.

Box 2.5: Using Kogler Hill's model in a primary healthcare nursing team

A team leader of an integrated primary healthcare nursing team was struggling to clarify her role leading to tensions within and outside the team. Using Kogler Hill's model as a framework, she worked through with her team what the model and associated elements meant in practice. The team were clearly able to see that in order for them to deliver optimum services, it was legitimate for her role to be both within and outside of the team. Moreover, this opportunity led the team to understand the degree to which effective teamworking is underpinned by task and relational aspects. The whole team used the complete framework to explore the team leader's and team members' roles and responsibilities, leading to greater clarity and less confusion.

As this chapter has suggested, much has been promised in terms of teamworking and linkages to positive impacts at a variety of levels, and some of this is reflected in research carried out in health and social care settings. However, many of these factors are not as clear-cut as the literature seems to suggest at first glance. There are a range of factors which help and hinder teamworking, some of which will be more applicable to some settings than others. It is important to remember that all organisations – and not just those within partnership settings – encounter a range of difficulties and challenges in attempting to forge more effective teams. Often these issues are not insurmountable, provided that the team has a clear focus on what it is aiming to achieve and how the strengths of the different members might be employed to meet those aims.

Reflective exercises

1. Consider three teams you have worked or played in. Make a list of all the positive and negative characteristics you think that these teams had.

2. Think about a team you enjoyed working in. What were the factors that made this enjoyable?

3. Think about a team you have not enjoyed working in. What were the factors that made this a negative experience and what did you do to overcome these issues?

4. For both the teams you thought about in response to the previous two questions, what factors hindered and what factors helped these teams? Are they similar to those suggested within this chapter?

5. Consider the organisation you are working in. What does it do to facilitate (or hinder) effective teamworking?

Further reading and resources

There are a range of web-based resources which offer evidence about the impacts of teamworking on performance and suggest how teamworking may be made more effective. A select few of these are suggested below:

• Aston Organisation Development (OD) is a spin-out company from Aston Business School that hosts a wealth of resources and information focused on the evidence around effective team-based working: www.astonod.com/index.php

• Research in Practice is the largest children and families research implementation project in England and Wales. Established in 1996 it is a department of the Dartington Hall Trust run in collaboration with the Association of Directors of Children's Services, the University of Sheffield and a network of over 100 participating agencies in the UK. Its mission is to promote positive outcomes for children and families through the use of research evidence: www. rip.org.uk

- Belbin Associates, home to the team building work of Meredith Belbin, is especially pertinent to roles in teams and includes resources and access to online team role inventories: www.belbin.com

- The NHS Institute for Innovation and Improvement has expertise in service transformation, technology and product innovation, leadership development and learning and has specific resources around effective teamworking: www.institute.nhs.uk

- The NHS Service Delivery and Organisation Research and Development Programme strives to produce and promote the use of research evidence about how the organisation and delivery of services can be improved to increase the quality of patient care, ensure better strategic outcomes and contribute to improved public health: www.sdo.lshtm.ac.uk/

For a more in-depth and critical discussion of IPE and leadership and management in partnership settings, see Carpenter and Dickinson (2008) and Peck and Dickinson (2008) in this series respectively.

Two meta-reviews of the teamworking literature that may be useful to draw on are one which focuses predominantly on healthcare by Borrill et al (2001), and one which draws more widely from commercial sector organisations by Parker and Bradley (2000).

3

Hot topics and emerging issues

This chapter explores a series of current hot topics and emerging issues associated with teamworking within interagency settings, including the following:

- As *communication* across organisational boundaries has been implicated as a major contributor to failures of safety in a number of high-profile cases, how can it be developed to ensure effectiveness in interagency settings?
- As improved *safety* is becoming an increasingly recognised tangible outcome of effective teamworking, what do teams need to do in order to develop a culture that improves safety for service users and staff?
- How can the changes and challenges of *decision making* and *devolution* within interagency settings be handled?

As suggested earlier, teamworking is a diverse field and the potential literature that may be drawn on is significant in both breadth and depth. Inevitably inclusion of these topics has meant we cannot talk in detail about other areas that may become increasingly important in the future (for example, self-managed teams and devolution). However, we have chosen to concentrate on these particular areas as we feel they are currently those most salient to health and social care teams and will likely remain central regardless of the rapidly shifting context in which we find ourselves. Moreover, in a number of cases it is difficult to be absolutely definitive about these issues. As suggested in Chapter 2, there are so many different factors that come into play when attempting to form effective interagency teams that much is contingent on the specific context of teams. In this chapter we attempt to draw together lessons from a diverse range of areas around these hot topics to supplement the authors' personal experiences. In Chapter 4 we then go on to present a range of frameworks that may be useful to employ – in both theoretical and practical terms – in attempting to form more effective teams.

Communication

Often the mere mention of the importance of communication and communication skills causes raised eyebrows, sighing and a shuffling of feet (Jelphs, 2006). We all use communication all the time – indeed, it is arguably imperative for our very survival on a day-to-day basis – yet communication is at the heart of many of the issues that have risen to prominence in relation to poor practice in health and social care and which have often had negative consequences for patients. Dunn et al (2007, p 213) highlight that this is a global issue, arguing that communication failure was involved in approximately 75% of more than 7,000 cause analysis reports to the Department of Veterans Affairs National Center for Patient Safety in the US. In the UK, the evidence from the Health and Social Care Information Service (2006) is clear: written and oral communication remain at the root of many of the complaints against health and social care services.

Much of what is written about communication in the fields of health and social care is predominantly concerned with the ways in which professionals, agencies and organisations interact. However, this often misses a key element of the jigsaw – the service user. In terms of written messages it is suggested that more attention needs to be paid to the literacy level of service users and that we should not assume that everyone has the same reading ability. If we define effective teamworking as really meeting the needs of service users it is sobering to reflect the extent of societal challenge in the UK with regards to literacy. For example, teams working with offenders – often across very complicated pathways and boundaries – need to consider that 80% have the writing skills, 65% the numeracy skills and 50% the reading skills at or below the level of an 11-year-old child (Home Office, 2002).

There are a range of issues that influence the sending and receiving of messages in everyday situations. Many of the points we make in this section are relatively straightforward or intuitive, but in the fast-paced environments of service delivery, elements of this best practice can become overlooked. One such point is that we cannot assume how others will interpret and act on (or whether they have the facilities to act on) any communications we make. A quote from the Victoria Climbié Inquiry illustrates this starkly: 'I cannot account for the way other people interpreted what I said. It was not the way I would have liked it to have been interpreted' (Laming, 2003, p 9). Although communication is often taken for granted as something we do all the time, effective communication is much more difficult to achieve in practice and involves not only the sending of a message, but its receipt and interpretation. Although we may think that we have said (or written) something that is relatively straightforward or comprehensible, there are a number of factors that influence whether this is the case, such as non-verbal communication, communication technologies, professional discourse, acronyms and abbreviations and international recruitment and language.

Non-verbal communication

Individual communication style is important and we are all different. In this book we argue that if teams are able to capitalise on the differences of their members, then they have the potential to be more effective. To do this, however, we need to invest time in exploring and understanding differences to harness these positively. In terms of spoken communication, one such factor is non-verbal communication (body language). Mehrabian (1972) suggests that this forms 70% of the message, whereas the words themselves are only 7% of the message and the tone of the delivery carries 23% of the message. This is well worth reflecting on and thinking about just how well we really know ourselves and our communication abilities. Often individuals have somewhat of a blind spot in relation to their ability to communicate effectively, and it is a useful exercise to think about how others might see and hear us.

As an example of the importance of such perceptions, commentators following the North American presidential election debate between Richard Nixon and John F. Kennedy speculated that if the event had not been televised and had simply been broadcast on the radio then Nixon may have won the debate. But in front of powerful television lights Nixon seemed uncomfortable next to Kennedy, who had taken advice on how to stand, what to wear and how to work with cameras. Nixon's words – and hence the content of the message – lost some of their power against Kennedy's considered, relaxed delivery style.

There are key learning points here, both in terms of the ways that we present ourselves and how this is in turn interpreted by others (and there are a number of overlaps in this argument with those of leadership and performance that are examined in *Managing and leading in inter-agency settings* by Edward Peck and Helen Dickinson in this series; readers interested in these issues may want to refer to this text for further discussion). There are also lessons here for those who are operating in multi- or interdisciplinary teams over multiple geographical locations. For health and social care teams, communication problems are often magnified by working in different locations, with diverse information systems that are not able to communicate with each other.

Communication technologies

We all form snap judgements about people as they do about us, and we need to reflect on how this can impact on our communication and relationships with others. Working across multiple sites may not necessarily impact negatively on communication between members, given the rise of different communication technologies and the use of video-conferencing facilities and so on. But in reality, access to and support to use these technologies varies enormously. As such, we need to pay close attention to the modes of communication that we use, and where and when these forms are and are not more suitable in comparison with others. Unlike the vast majority of acute services, not all staff members working in the community can easily access computer and printer facilities. There are undoubtedly major systemic issues that need investing in if teamworking is to be as effective as possible and these do not always mean spending large amounts of money. Investing small sums and empowering teams to be able to spend wisely will make a real difference.

A number of partnership evaluations have cited IT as a major barrier to interorganisational information sharing and this has proved to be a major barrier to partnership working (Richardson and Asthana, 2005). A Department of Health report found that the information aspects of partnership working lag well behind the general state of partnership working (Rhodes, 2003). These problems may include legal information-sharing barriers, difficulties with incompatible IT systems or a lack of common referral systems (Cameron and Lart, 2003). However, simply improving information systems or using them more extensively will not necessarily produce more effective communication or teamwork. Although it is clearly important that professionals are able to communicate well, and information technologies aid this to an extent (particularly when teams are not co-located), it is a myth that by simply getting this right teams will be able to function effectively, just as it is a myth that by structuring organisations/teams in the 'right' way they will automatically be more successful.

Indeed, there is some research suggesting that IT can cause its own difficulties, such as the growth of email as a form of communication. Bevan (2006) suggests that NHS leaders fit the pattern identified by recent research across business sectors: that is, struggling to stay on top of a torrent of unfocused and unnecessary emails, which can mean that important priorities are often hidden or missed. However, staff need not be passive recipients of this deluge. It is really worth investing some time to develop systems for using email (and other communication systems) that individuals and teams are comfortable with. A team one of the authors worked with recently identified the following actions:

- stop irrelevant email and paper duplication;
- consider whether the email relevant to everybody;
- think about the clarity of the title of the email;
- think about junk emails and the organisational systems;

- consider small group emails and their use;
- consider a flag system to code information.

None of this is rocket science, but this large multidisciplinary team recognised that addressing this issue was vital and devoted time at an away day to agree practical actions, including exploring personal responsibility and negotiating with the organisation about some of the wider systems and processes (for further discussion, see Jelphs, 2006).

Professional discourse and communication

The majority of the Labour government's attempts to promote and improve partnership working have focused on policies, processes and structures, rather than on the individuals and professionals who are actually interacting with one another. In other words, the focus on interorganisational working has not been matched by equal attention to interprofessional relationships (Hudson, 2002). As we have suggested, simply getting the structures and technologies of partnerships 'right' (whatever that may entail) does not mean that we will get productive and effective interagency teams. Much sociological research has suggested that professions are essentially self-interested groupings. As such, professionals are socialised into these groups and holding a particular professional identity can become a valued part of an individual's personal identity (Evetts, 1999).

The process of professional training not only passes on 'official' learning in the sense of the technical skills with which professionals are imbued, but also serves to institutionalise professionals into certain ways of acting and thinking. That is, individuals become part of a particular professional discourse that provides a social boundary that defines what can be said about a specific topic, or what might be considered the limits of acceptable speech (for a practical example of this within mental health services, see 6 et al, 2007). This discourse impacts not only on what it is possible to say, but also on the ways in which communications are made. For example, social workers have very clear ideas of what they understand by supervision and what good supervision means, which is often different to the supervision experienced and expected by health colleagues. Similarly, nurses tend to be trained to speak in a narrative way, whereas doctors tend to focus on precise facts. This is now changing, but if both doctors and nurses are socialised into communicating in these ways and recognise that this way of communicating is acceptable, then there are going to be difficulties when trying to communicate in new structured ways.

Different professions and professionals will – to a certain extent – all have their own languages and will have been socialised – or educated – into specific ways of seeing and accepting the world. When others do not interpret or understand the world in the same way there is potential for real conflict and individuals can feel isolated, especially if they have the minority view in a team. The degree of difference between professional discourses will impact on and shape interprofessional relations. Where members of a profession have similar perceptions, values and experiences they will likely be more in agreement than with members of a different profession. It is this degree of difference in these values, perceptions and experiences that will influence how professions interact. However, differences do not just occur between professions, and a number of issues (for example, geographical location, specialism, leadership style) may form differences *within* professions. In this case, professionals may find that they have more in common with individuals from other professions who are working within a similar context to themselves.

By understanding that different professionals think and communicate in different ways and find different forms of information acceptable, individuals may find that they react differently to communication with other professions. Rather than reacting in an aggressive way, individuals may have a better comprehension of why professionals are communicating in different ways and try to overcome these rather than dismissing out of hand information that does not fit their particular discourse. Sheehan et al (2007) argue that there are distinct differences in the sophistication of communication between multidisciplinary and interprofessional teams. Their research identified that multidisciplinary team members worked and communicated in parallel ways, not really sharing or considering the wider significance of specific information, whereas interprofessional teams demonstrated a more inclusive language, were more collaborative and continually shared information. Interprofessional teams tried to create their own language, one that was acceptable and understood by the different professions.

Just as professionals accept and reject certain types of information, so too do service users. The way in which professionals interact and communicate with service users will, to a certain extent, determine the degree to which individuals take messages on board and act in terms of their care. Some professionals try hard to use inclusive language and be as clear with service users as possible, but as Box 3.1 illustrates, while this is often appreciated by service users, it may not be as popular with other professionals who may feel that their specialism is being undermined. But it is not just the use of these terms in the spoken word that needs attention. The Health Service Ombudsmen lamented in 2004, 'if only all health service staff made sure they listened to patients and their carers, communicated clearly with them and with each other, then made a note of what had been said, the scope for later misunderstanding and dispute would be reduced enormously' (*British Medical Journal*, 2004, p 10).

Box 3.1: Using language in a way to include service users

A consultant surgeon found himself isolated and often teased by colleagues for his approach to working with patients to get consent forms signed. He deliberately explained the operating procedure in everyday language supported by diagrams and used the same words on the consent forms – so patients were absolutely clear what they were consenting to. He was passionate that this approach was needed to reinforce communication and was the key to working in partnership with patients to get informed consent. However, he was disheartened that the approach was not respected by many of his colleagues, highlighting just how hard it can be for professionals to challenge accepted procedures in order to develop more patient-centred services. In this case, it was perhaps because it was perceived by some colleagues that some of the mystique of professional language associated with maintaining professionalism would be reduced.

Acronyms and abbreviations

Communication difficulties are further compounded by a propensity to use acronyms. The fields of health and social care are replete with the use of a wide range of acronyms and abbreviations that are not necessarily understood by all, particularly when some abbreviations have multiple meanings. This is especially important for teams working across boundaries and agencies who often use similar acronyms for completely different things, compounding confusion and often alienating people from discussions. Not only does this need to be challenged by professionals, but if service users are to have access to their records they must be able to understand them and using a plethora of acronyms and abbreviations might prove problematic.

International recruitment and language

If teams do not pay attention to language and meaning and develop systems and processes which are agreed and understood by all, it is likely that they will not function as well as they could. One very practical issue that both health and social care are currently facing is the use of international recruitment to enhance the workforce. There is an issue over whether teams are really spending time understanding the impact of different languages and cultures on their colleagues and the wider team, or whether they are being encouraged to do this at all. It seems that there is often an assumption that these individuals will have to adapt so that they will fit in, rather than teams adapting to take account of this diversity of language, culture and experience. Box 3.2 gives an example of a team made of individuals from a number of different countries and the impact that their cultures had on the effectiveness of the team.

Box 3.2: Overseas recruitment and team effectiveness

A large multicultural forensic unit team with members from the Caribbean, Far East, India, Eastern Europe and UK was struggling to work effectively. The unit manager recognised that the team were struggling and from conversations with the service director and individual team members it became clear that there were major differences in interpreting and understanding the underlying philosophy of the unit, often resulting in impassioned debate and confusion around care delivery. When the team took time out together and stopped to look at why there was increasing conflict, they realised that their socialisation to different cultural approaches and working practices towards forensic mental health were very different.

For some team members a rehabilitative approach was an alien concept. As the rationale for working in this way, together with expected staff behaviours, had not been fully communicated (or understood), they struggled with care delivery in the unit. Time out as a team gave individuals the opportunity to share their experiences and concerns, which predominantly related to under-standing their philosophies of care and expectations of working in teams. It was agreed that the whole team needed to clearly understand and commit to a vision and philosophy, and needed to invest time to enhance relationships and communication. This was done by the director leading a session around philosophy and achievements that they were particularly proud of, together with a more structured approach around team meetings, support and supervision. The key lesson learnt was not to assume that new team members automatically understood what the team was trying to achieve, and that it was important to realise that their challenges were helpful in ensuring the team was constantly reflecting on itself and practice. Crucially, other team members further understood that teamworking could mean many different things in other countries, with different expectations of individual members, and different approaches to working with hierarchy and taking responsibility. As a result of these interventions and ongoing support, relationships and consistency of care improved.

—

But, as Box 3.2 illustrates, perhaps the most important thing in terms of communication is that teams need *time*. There is real evidence that teams that take time to meet and use their time wisely are more effective. West and Markiewcz (2004, p 106) argue that the whole point of teamwork is the bringing together of people with different experiences, skills and knowledge to achieve a task that is better met by a group, which means high levels of participation is key. This is a real issue as many large teams struggle to find the space for all team members to meet together. Organisations and managers must therefore consider the practical needs of teams when developing estates and/or training and development strategies. Furthermore as virtual, distributed and home working for teams grows, the very real issue of where people are going to meet to talk and listen to each other becomes ever more fundamental.

Safety

There is a growing interest in and literature on the importance of teamworking in enhancing safety for patients, service users, carers and staff. For those sceptical about the claims of teamworking, safety may eventually become the key that persuades people that investment in these processes is really worthwhile. Learning from other sectors may be useful in this respect and there has been much research from commercial industry that this section will draw on.

High-reliability organisations

There is a substantial literature relating to 'high-reliability' organisations – typically such organisations as power grid despatching centres, nuclear power generating plants, air traffic controllers, hostage negotiation teams, Navy nuclear aircraft carriers and hospital emergency teams. In each of these organisations the concept of failure is absolutely central. The concept of reliability is essentially a non-dynamic event. In other words, reliable systems try their hardest to maintain a status where there are no adverse events (failures), while accepting that human variability is inevitable. In the activities of the industries outlined above it is vital that non-event states are maintained in their activities (Weick, 1987). The aim of these organisations is to deliver a consistent performance in the face of disruptive change and volatility in the business environment. Such organisations have to establish systems through which they can avoid moments of misperception or lack of attention so that minor failures do not escalate into unmanageable difficulties. High-reliability organisations must avoid weak responses even when faced by signals that seem relatively innocuous. These organisations aim to achieve stability of performance by means of constant change and mutual adjustments, so that the impact of the unexpected becomes a dynamic non-event (Ojha, 2005).

One such example is that provided by Firth-Cozens (2001), who comments on and summarises research into fatigue in aircraft flight crews. Crews who were tired, but who had flown together for several days, were found to make fewer errors than crews who were not tired but who had not worked together for so long. It is suggested that team members were able to compensate for the errors of their colleagues through recognising when things were going wrong and being able to coordinate or compensate effectively. Or, perhaps, effective teamworking meant that stress levels were already lower in these crews compared to the others in the study. This suggests that stability is an important issue for health and social care teams to consider. This is especially pertinent where there is a climate of short-term contracts and widespread use of agency staff, which have the potential to mitigate against such stability. As suggested earlier, links between effective teamworking and reduced stress levels are growing within the research literature. When people are stressed they often make small mistakes, find their memory is not so good, or feel unwell and narrow down their focus of attention as a way of coping. These are all valid coping mechanisms, but a consequence is that individuals find they have less time for the views and thoughts of others and are not so aware of the environment around them.

'Safe' cultures

Creating 'safe' cultures is not just about creating a team culture that focuses on the issue of safety (as a number of the high-reliability organisations outlined above do). It is also about creating a team that has shared commitment to its overall goals and clarity that individuals are accountable not just for their own contribution but for the quality of the service the whole team delivers. Such a culture means that there is a greater shared interest in the service provided and suggests that individuals have a duty of care to speak up when things are going wrong. In order for individuals to report something if things are going wrong there needs to be a climate where people feel safe to do this. Although the concept of a 'no blame culture' is often referred to in health and social care, we think that a 'safe' culture is perhaps more useful. Such safe cultures are ones where people can trust one another and are treated justly. Undeniably, at times people do need to be held accountable for their errors, but within safe cultures is it important that they are, and are seen to be, treated fairly in response to these issues.

In situations where there are punitive measures in response to reported incidents or 'near-misses', teams may find there are much fewer incidents actually reported than in situations where such reports lead to investigations into the real root causes of these events. As Leape (1994, p 1851) identifies, 'ironically, rather than improving safety, punishment makes reducing errors much more difficult by providing strong incentives for people to hide their mistakes, thus preventing recognition, analysis and correction of underlying cause'. Organisations must mean it when they say that they need to learn from errors if learning is to impact positively on safety in the future. Quality theorist W. Edwards Deming (quoted in Seddon, 2004) estimates that 95% of the cause of variation in performance is attributable to the system that the work of a team is structured around. In other words, he suggests that failure is due to the way the work is designed and managed, rather than necessarily the people executing the tasks. This might be an overstatement in terms of the importance of structure and process, but most organisational theorists would agree that most significant breakdowns in safety are not purely the result of the actions of an inattentive individual(s), but relate to other systemic influences.

In a study of incident reporting in children's services, Bostock et al (2005) argue that we will only be better able to learn how to protect children and young people if we look at so-called near-misses as well as at incidents of serious harm. In other words, while traditionally in health and social care incidents are reported when they have led to some form of harm being caused to children and families, the research team worked with children's services who piloted 'safeguarding incidents'. These incidents cover everything that could have or did cause harm to children and families. This process tends to actually focus on the 'no harm' incidents or near-misses as research shows that learning from these types of 'free mistakes' might actually prevent more serious incidents in the future. Just as high-reliability organisations capture a wealth of information about potential near-misses, if child welfare organisations were to adapt such an approach this would 'reveal weaknesses in the necessarily complex assessment, decision-making and review systems surrounding child welfare and show ways of correcting them' (Bostock et al, 2005, p xiii). In other words, by creating a more open culture where professionals are encouraged to report potential incidents then organisational learning is much greater and serious incidents are less likely to occur.

Much is spoken about a learning culture, and it looks set to be another buzzword of organisational theory. But what is it really? A learning culture is one where people are interested in understanding what has happened, why it happened and take steps to ensure that it does not happen again. Moreover, learning organisations share their learning and experiences widely in order to prevent errors and enhance safety (as seen in the case of high-reliability organisations above). Health and social care agencies are starting to do this, but have a long way to go to catch up with airlines who have an advanced system for sharing lessons across diverse and often competing organisations (see, for example, Hamman, 2004).

It is perhaps helpful at this point to focus more on the concepts of learning and organisations. Edmonson (1999) argues that organisational learning is defined in two different ways in the literature, with some authors discussing learning as an outcome, and others focusing on a process they define as learning. Edmonson identifies that she is clearly in the second camp (1999, p 353) and her research attempts to articulate behaviours through which outcomes such as adapting to change, developing greater understanding or increasing performance in teams can take place (which she calls learning behaviour). Different approaches to learning are further illuminated by introducing models of single and double-loop learning and by highlighting the differences in approach and possible significance for health and social care. Single-loop learning is characterised as adaptive learning, which focuses on how to improve the status quo (Argyris and Schön, 1978) and may:

- lead to a situation of individuals questioning 'whose fault it was' and therefore seemingly apportioning blame;
- engender a culture of fear and anxiety about making mistakes;
- potentially lead to a concealment of errors;
- tackle the obvious problem, but not necessarily the underlying cause.

Double-loop learning takes a generative, more enquiring approach to learning that is aimed at changing the status quo and can potentially lead to transformational change. Double-loop learning is:

- driven by a constant desire for improvement;
- encourages openness around mistakes and errors;
- nurtures a climate of trust and responsibility;
- invests in finding the cause of the problem as well as the symptoms;
- is ultimately interested in understanding why something happened in order to prevent it happening again;
- focuses on individual, team and organisational levels.

For this reason, double-loop learning has been suggested to hold the potential to offer much to health and social care improvement programmes. Figure 3.1 illustrates single and double-loop learning in a graphical format.

Figure 3.1: Single and double-loop learning

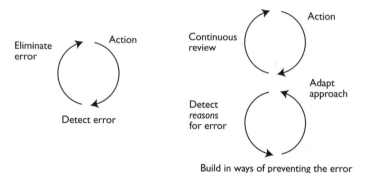

Source: Adapted from Argyris and Schön (1978)

Edmonson (1999, p 354) argues that teams need to develop psychological safety, which she defines as 'a shared belief that the team is safe for interpersonal risk taking'. The creation of a safe environment is crucial if people are to have the confidence to speak up when things go wrong. Individuals need to feel secure and know that they will not be victimised for speaking up, but developing the confidence to do so means that there must be mutual trust and respect among team members. It is crucial to highlight here that trust does not develop easily or quickly; it takes time and therefore the issue of the need for stability in teams arises again.

Edmonson's work on medication errors in North American hospitals again adds valuable insights (1996). She identified that leader behaviour was fundamental in developing a climate whereby mistakes and errors could be discussed safely and openly. Teams run in a dictatorial or hierarchical fashion were less likely to report errors than those that were more horizontally organised with distributed leadership. Additionally she identified what many others know intuitively, that where there is a climate of trust and openness, reporting of errors may initially rise. It is crucial that team leaders understand this so they understand the initial consequences of developing a culture where people are not

—

afraid to share and disclose errors and mistakes. As an example of this, in 2006 figures indicated that the number of racially motivated crimes recorded by police in England and Wales went up by 12% (Home Office, 2006). However, rather than suggesting this was negative and indicated an increase in racist incidents, the Association of Chief Police Officers (ACPO) suggested the rise was in part an indication of the success of work done to encourage victims of such crimes to come forward. In other words, ACPO suggested this rise in reporting illustrated a culture that has become better aware and more sensitive to these kinds of offences. It is also important to recognise that some teams have two leaders, especially if there are members from different organisations or agencies (or perhaps teams have one leader but report to different managers). A lack of consistency and different behaviours in relation to supporting staff that have made or disclosed errors will be very divisive and mitigate against real teamworking. Figure 3.2 illustrates the type of trend we might expect to see in the reporting of near-misses when trying to form a more open culture.

Figure 3.2: Expected pattern for near-miss reporting in creating a more open culture

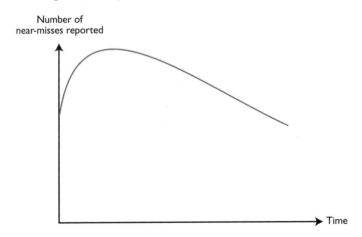

Decision making and devolution

This section explores the issue of decision making in further detail as the authors' experience is that this remains a hot topic, especially for teams working in and across complex environments. Cook et al (2001) argue that this very complexity should not automatically be considered problematic, as it might provide new opportunities for different ways of making decisions. In fact they go on to argue that if teams are able to develop autonomy, they are better able to orientate decisions to meet the needs of service users. However, a consequence of this may be that existing orientations of service provision are challenged, or even threatened, which can lead to people outside the team being marginalised as active participants in decision making. Katzenbach and Smith (1993) argue that 'real' teams are the ones that are decisive and in control. They accept that this takes time to develop and assert that there is a delicate balancing act to be undertaken by a team's leader with regards to decision making. As Øvretveit (1995, p 43) argues, 'the right decision-making process is critical for using different professionals' expertise to the best effect and for energy, morale and work satisfaction in teams'.

Categories of decision making

Macdonald (1990) suggests that there are four major categories of decision making. Which approach is employed depends on the type of problem that is being addressed, the range of information available to the decision maker and the nature of the situation. These different approaches are outlined as:

- *rational:* goal-centred, logical and efficient;
- *consensual:* demand participation with general agreement, have bias towards democratic;
- *empirical:* based on information and evidence, demands credibility;
- *political:* focus and reliance on adaptability to situation.

Arguably, all of these approaches could be legitimate at any given time, depending on the nature of the issue or problem being addressed. Much of the partnership literature argues that teams should veer towards the consensual model in the interests of democracy and a preference to avoid argument and heated debate (more of which later). But clearly, the way in which a decision is made will depend on the type of decision that is being made and within what timeframe. Consensual, democratic models of decision making would suggest that, ideally, as many team members as possible need to be involved in both decision making and decision taking. But at times it is just not feasible, or arguably necessary, to involve everyone. Team decision making does not mean that everyone has to be involved in every decision. What is crucial is that teams have an agreed process for decision making, and within that process there is clarity and understanding about when, how and who will (or needs to be) involved. However, just making the decision is only part of the process. Clutterbuck (2007) argues that unless decision making is supported by an understanding of what the decision means, together with an individual and collective commitment to take it forward, it is valueless (see Figure 3.3) (this is further explored in the model of team dysfunction in Chapter 4).

Figure 3.3: Commitment, understanding and decision making

	Low commitment and understanding	High commitment and understanding
Good decision	Benefits lost through poor implementation	Rapid and effective implementation
Poor decision	Confusion	Rapid implementation of the wrong thing

Source: Clutterbuck (2007)

—

Whose decision?

Some teams struggle with understanding and being comfortable with accountability for decision making and believe that only the team leader, or most senior person, is accountable. However, as the General Medical Council (2006) suggests about the position of consultant psychiatrists working in multidisciplinary teams, referrals are made directly to such teams and decisions about allocation to an appropriate professional are made according to the teams' policies. In these teams, the responsibility for the care of patients is distributed among the clinical members of the team. Consultants retain oversight of a group of patients who are allocated to their care and are responsible for providing advice and support to the team. They are not accountable for the actions of other clinicians in the team. As Øvretveit (1995) suggests, it is perhaps more helpful for managers and team members to be clear about responsibilities in order for there to be workable, understood decision-making procedures.

The notion of transparency about role responsibility is thus useful in clarifying concerns about accountability. Many concerns about working across boundaries reflect the perception (and often reality) that certain professionals have more power over decision making and that challenging those professionals is problematic (reflecting some of the barriers highlighted in Table 3.1). Without stereotyping it is true to say that doctors are often assumed to be in this category. However, research by Gair and Hartley (2001) contradicts the notion that doctors always dominate discussions. Their research found that doctors were more likely to have their proposals questioned and were willing to accept decisions contrary to their initial suggestions. This raises the question of behavioural responses to challenges, which is considered further below. As we have stated throughout this text it is important to remember that teams are part of a wider system and this impacts on decision-making processes. Organisations that are supportive of teamworking will ensure that there is clarity over boundaries of the decisions that the teams (and their leaders) are able and expected to take, and commit to those agreed boundaries, unlike the example in Box 3.3.

Box 3.3: Devolved decision making and the wider system

As part of an ongoing process to develop self-managed teams and devolution in a primary care trust (PCT), budgetary responsibility had been devolved to integrated community nursing teams. The teams were clear about the specific elements that appeared in the budget statements and one team decided to purchase new uniforms (the money was in the budget), their rationale being that they wanted all team members to wear the same uniform in an attempt to reduce hierarchical associations with different uniforms (name badges would clearly state names and roles). Their purchase order was stopped because the director of nursing did not want different uniforms to be worn by different teams. The consequence of this was very poor relationships between the team and the PCT, with the team refusing to be involved in further decision making over budgetary issues. A key lesson for organisations here is that if you are going to devolve decision making, be prepared to live with difference and be clear what the boundaries are.

Rational, social and behavioural perspectives

Adair (1997) argues that there is a classic five-step approach to decision making: define the objective, collect relevant information, generate feasible options, make the decision and implement it, and evaluate. This is both a rational and logical approach to decision making, but the reality is often much more confused and messy. Much of the literature identifies that social and behavioural perspectives need to be recognised if we are to acknowledge that individual weaknesses and bias can inhibit taking a rational approach to decision making (if a rational approach is at all possible). If the logic behind developing teams is that collectively they will achieve more, then it follows that, collectively, teams should make better decisions than individuals. However, the evidence challenges this notion. Although teams do make better decisions than the average team member, it is suggested that often the decisions are not of the same quality as that which the

—

Table 3.1: Barriers to effective decision making in teams

Process	Effect
Personality factors	May inhibit social behaviour, for example team members who are shy may struggle to contribute to the discussion
Social conformity	Possible withholding of opinion and information that is contrary to the majority view
Lack of communication skills	Individuals may struggle to present opinions, knowledge and views successfully
Dominance by individuals	May monopolise a lot of discussion time or use their personality to override the views of others in a forceful way
Egocentric members	Team members may be unwilling to consider the views, experiences and opinions of others – may (but not necessarily) be in senior positions
Status and hierarchy	May unduly influence the group through their position – contributions can be valued in a disproportionate manner
Risky shift	Propensity for groups to make more extreme decisions – may be more risky or more conservative
Group think	Irving Janis (1972) identified that groups may be more concerned with maintaining group cohesiveness and agreement than making an uncomfortable decision. A number of investigations into public disasters and major events have identified this factor as contributing to the poor quality of decisions made. Group think arises as a result of the desire to minimise conflict, but often at the expense of thinking critically or testing these ideas. This may arise as individuals do not want to look foolish, or because it is so important that a group remains cohesive that individual doubts are set aside (however valid they may be). The NASA spaceship Challenger disaster and the Cuban Bay of Pigs affair are two high profile examples found in the literature (for further information on these events, see, respectively, Vaughan, 1996; Allison and Zelikow, 1999)
Social loafing	Individuals may work less hard if they believe their contribution is masked by the rest of the team
Diffusion of responsibility	Individuals assume responsibility for action should be taken by others

Source: Adapted from West and Markiewicz (2004, p 110)

—

best individual team member could make (West and Markiewicz, 2004). One of the real values in teams making decisions together is the collective ownership this involvement facilitates, which should lead to a greater commitment to implement the outcome. Therefore, as we have consistently suggested, teams are complex social entities and are potentially prey to social processes that can undermine their decision-making procedures. West and Markiewcz (2004, p 110) have summarised barriers to effective decision making in teams (adapted in Table 3.1).

Conflict

A number of the barriers outlined in Table 3.1 have been produced out of a desire to avoid conflict. However, conflict is not necessarily negative (although it is often assumed to be), and may actually have positive impacts on teamworking. Conflict can be defined as occurring where the concerns of two people *appear* to be incompatible. Conflict arises because essentially people see the world differently, and how that difference manifests itself in behaviour can be why conflict has so many negative associations for many people. But if teams are to be effective they need to find ways of positively working with difference (see the following section for more on this). The Thomas Kilman model of conflict handling (Thomas, 2002) is based on a person's behaviour along two basic dimensions:

- *assertiveness:* the extent to which the individual attempts to satisfy her/his own concerns;
- *cooperativeness:* the extent to which the individual attempts to satisfy the other person's concerns.

Figure 3.4 describes five specific methods of dealing with conflicts that individuals may adopt:

- *accommodation:* help another individual or group achieve their goals, but often at the expense of reaching your own;
- *collaboration:* work with other individuals or groups to achieve their goals and yours;

Figure 3.4: Thomas Kilman's (2002) model of managing conflict

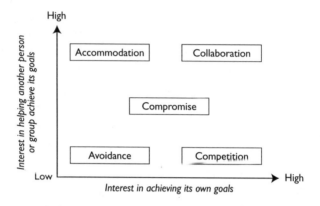

- *compromise:* middle ground where everybody compromises and only achieves some of their goals;
- *avoidance:* does not reach either their own goals or those of other individuals or groups. Is uncooperative and unassertive;
- *competition:* will pursue their own goals at the expense of other individuals or groups reaching their goals.

Although much of the partnership working literature identifies collaboration as a main objective, other behavioural styles may also be justifiable dependent on the situation and the task(s) that the specific partnership is faced with achieving. Partnerships may wish to think about where the interests of their agency and those of their partners lie on this matrix and which models of managing conflict are most appropriate.

Working with diversity

Many studies have identified that diversity in team membership and working across boundaries can impact positively on performance and decision making (for examples of such studies, see Jackson et al, 1991 and also Box 3.4).

Box 3.4: The value of diversity in decision making

Some nursing members of a multidisciplinary community mental health team were struggling to manage their caseload. The effect of this was that they did not have the capacity to take on new referrals, which had an impact on the workloads of other team members, resulting in increasingly strained relationships. Discussion with the wider team showed part of their reluctance to discharge people against the established criteria was a fear of making the wrong decision. It was decided that nursing team members would pair up for supervision with social workers. This worked exceptionally well as the skills and experiences of the social workers, together with their different ways of 'seeing situations', helped allay fears, and nurses were able to discharge with more confidence.

However, it has also been suggested that there are a maximum number of diverse views above which decision making becomes too protracted and difficult. Øvretveit (1995, p 42) argues that teams sometimes try to minimise differences and it is perhaps helpful to illuminate his assertions as they are useful in explaining some of the very real issues which impact on teamworking in health and social care:

- Teams are fearful that differences will be too destructive on team functioning.
- Practitioners have some skills and knowledge in common, which are often seen by professional associations as unique to individual professions, leading practitioners to perhaps fear that national battles could erupt in the team and lead to competition for valued work.
- Some team members wish to defend hard-won autonomy and fear that if differences in skill and expertise emerge and come to be seen as more important in the team, the consequence could be that one or more professions becomes more dominant, with others losing autonomy.

- Minimising differences is congruent with developing more equal relationships with clients and therefore equality is encouraged while status symbols and power displays are reduced.

All these seem like legitimate responses when faced by potentially difficult and stressful situations. However, diversity brings different perspectives, experiences and ways of seeing the world and as such may contribute to passionate and heated debate. Under some circumstances we might encourage this, as teams which do not have lively, impassioned debates may be trying too hard to maintain cohesiveness and hence move to a model of 'group think' (Janis, 1972). A substantial proportion of the partnership literature continually re-iterates the importance of harmonious relationships and avoiding undue conflict. However, if team members do not challenge practices or decisions within partnership settings, they may find that they seriously compromise the quality of their decision making.

Working across boundaries

A salient point for team members, especially those working across boundaries, is how decision making is recorded and communicated (and this links into an earlier hot topic). Differences in professional training, socialisation and therefore expectations of other professionals with regards to record keeping and the clear documentation of decisions and actions can potentially lead to angst and uncertainty. Single patient records may assist teams up to a point, but they will only be as good as their content and how it is determined and acted on. Furthermore, people who cross boundaries and are part of decision-making processes in other agencies or organisations must have the necessary authority and autonomy to contribute to discussions, problem solving and decision making, along with the confidence to participate fully. They need to believe, and other team members need to recognise that, they have legitimacy of presence. Figure 3.5 encapsulates the interdependence needed between different elements: *autonomy* is about having the authority to act in a certain context; *influence* is related to having the

Figure 3.5: Decision making across boundaries

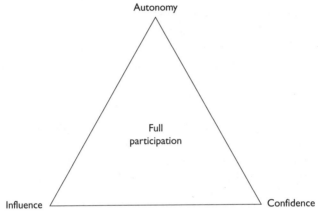

ability and skill to shape the situation; and *confidence* reflects feelings and the need for positive emotion in taking part.

This section has demonstrated that decision making in teams is a complex concept and there are no easy answers for all situations – team members need to pay close attention to the nature of the problem that they are addressing, the risk that this decision entails, which stakeholders need to be involved and so forth.

In this chapter we have already outlined some frameworks that may aid professionals in these difficult processes. The next chapter outlines a further range of frameworks and concepts which will be useful for teams operating in interagency settings to draw on and which will offer suggestions for more effective working.

Reflective exercises

In response to these questions think about a team you are a member of. If you are not a member of a team presently, think of a time in the past when you have been a member of a work team, or else, think of a team that you have been a member of in your personal life or a team you have read about.

1. Take time to consider communication in your 'home' team (the work team you spend most time with). What image or metaphor would you use to describe the reality of communication? What does this tell you about communication in your team, and, importantly, what improvements would you like to see?

2. The next time you meet a new person take time to reflect on what judgements you make about them and why. Then take time to consider what judgements they may have made about you.

3. Think about a map that shows the community of teams that your team interacts with. Do you share messages and learning (from errors, complaints and compliments) with all?

4. Consider the single and double-looped learning model illustrated in this chapter. Which model reflects practice in your team?

5. Reflect on an adverse incident that has taken place in a team you have experience of. What did you think, what did you feel and what did you do in this situation?

6. Imagine your team is sitting around a table where decisions are being made. Looking in on this situation, what behaviours and skills do you see?

7. Consider Table 3.1. How many of these apply to decisions made by the team(s) you are working in and what were the consequences?

Further reading and resources

This chapter has covered a broad range of issues, and readers may want to follow up specific topics in more detail. As a result, the further reading and resources below are necessarily diverse to enable people to explore all the issues that are relevant to them and their local context.

- The National Patient Safety Agency aims to put patient safety at the top of the NHS agenda through encouraging greater transparency and accountability for the provision of safer healthcare in all settings. The website contains useful tools and frameworks including an e-learning, multimedia package that has seven modules, including one on teamworking: www.npsa.nhs.uk

- For practical advice, support and resources for improving meetings, including presentation skills see www.effectivemeetings.com or www.meetingwizard.org

- The Institute for Healthcare Improvement website hosts a wealth of evidence-based information and tools aimed at improving and enhancing understanding of effective care delivery. These have been designed to offer easy, convenient access to quality experts and cutting-edge content: www.ihi.org

- For further exploration of communication issues see Stanton's (2003) *Mastering communication*.

- The Social Care Institute for Excellence report by Bostock et al (2005), *Managing risk and minimising mistakes to services for children and families*, may be a useful resource in aiding professionals to think through how they could better report near-misses and produce organisational learning that avoids major incidents.

- For further detail on decision making see the National Co-ordinating Centre for NHS Service Delivery and Organisation Research and Development's (2001) report *Making informed decisions on change – Key points for health care managers and professionals*.

4

Useful frameworks and concepts

Throughout this book we have tried to convey the message that just concentrating on individual teams is not enough in the complex world of health and social care delivery. Much of the text so far has been concerned with problematising the nature of teams and teamworking and the impacts that this may have for partnership working. Historically, much effort has gone into developing single teams, while not perhaps recognising or paying enough attention to the environment that teams operate within. This chapter aims to introduce a range of models, frameworks and tools that have been successfully tried and tested in teams working in and across a variety of organisational settings. Some are examples from the established private sector and or health/social care literature, while others are new and innovative approaches used by the authors. Models and frameworks are sometimes perceived as only having academic relevance, but they are a way of representing the reality of the world and can help in making sense of what sometimes seem overwhelmingly complex situations and issues (while acknowledging that models are not inevitably direct reflections of the world we live in). The models and frameworks in this chapter have been chosen to help structure thinking and work around teams, to increase understanding and, perhaps, to highlight where effort and resources may be best targeted when attempting to build and develop effective teams and associated partnerships.

The chapter starts by introducing a model that captures the critical dimensions of multidisciplinary working (Figure 4.1), and demonstrates the various internal factors that are important in creating effective teams. This is then followed by another model that highlights the interdependent elements needed for effective partnership working

– the *effective partnership working inventory* (West and Markiewicz, 2006) – which outlines the major themes to concentrate on when trying to get different teams to work together more effectively (see Figure 4.2). The seven individual dimensions of the inventory then guide the structure and presentation of the rest of the chapter and consist of:

- shared commitment to goals and objectives
- interdependence of outcomes
- role clarity
- cultural congruity
- focus on quality and innovation
- true cooperation
- interprofessional trust and respect.

Each dimension will be supported by a range of frameworks, models and tools that we hope will be understandable, practical and easy to use. The further reading and resources section at the end of this chapter has been designed to signpost to a wide range of tools to complement this material.

Critical dimensions of multidisciplinary working

Gorman (1998) suggests that structure, interprofessional relationships and processes are critical to effective multidisciplinary working. Gorman produced a model of these processes, which the model in Figure 4.1 is based on. What Figure 4.1 suggests is that teams need to pay attention to structures, processes and culture as they will all impact and influence behaviours, which (as we have seen) can either facilitate effective teamworking or act as a major barrier. It is perhaps helpful to explain in more detail what these three areas mean and, importantly, how they manifest themselves.

In terms of the *structural* issues that are important in creating effective interagency teams, factors include:

- *Geography/location:* there is very good evidence that teams who are based together are likely, but not necessarily able, to work together more effectively. Often lack of a shared location is suggested as the

---

78

Figure 4.1: Critical dimensions of multidisciplinary working

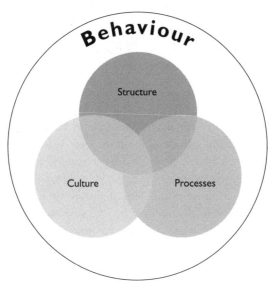

main reason that teams were not able to work together effectively. However, it does not automatically follow that just because teams are co-located they will interact better (for such an example, see Davey et al, 2005), and process and interpersonal factors will need to be considered in tangent.

- *Different employers:* many teams work for different employers (for example, NHS trusts, GPs, voluntary agencies, local authorities etc) with their associated employment practices, policies and procedures, and this is a major challenge. Although it is potentially easier if all members work for one employer, committed effective teams can work with and around differences in a positive way.

- *Accountability:* confusion over accountability is a major hindrance to effective teamworking. In multidisciplinary teams, team members are usually accountable for their work to the team leader (who may be of a different discipline) and will be accountable professionally to a

—

leader who may not be based in the team. Confusion arises when systems are not clear and support is perceived as insufficient.

- *Failure to clarify systems of working:* when teams integrate, this is a major area of unrest and deserves significant attention to remove duplication and parallel systems that hinder effective working.

- *Allegiances:* some areas of health and social care have identified concerns from employers that team members who have different employers will have a loyalty to that employer. Having an allegiance to an organisation outside of the team a professional works in is sometimes seen as problematic and is perceived to hinder effective multidisciplinary teamworking. For example, some GPs have suggested that, for example, district nurses, health visitors and school nurses who are employed by PCTs will adhere to specific organisational systems and processes that may inhibit their ability to tailor their actions to meet the differing population needs of their practice.

As we have continually re-iterated throughout this text, sorting out these structural issues alone will not result in effective teams. Moreover, as we have previously noted, these difficulties are not simply restricted to partnerships but are encountered by other types of organisations. It is also important to note that some of these factors are linked. In terms of interpersonal/behavioural issues, poor relationships are the biggest cause of work-based stress and working in a team that is not working well impacts on the individuals directly involved, and the wider team. Attention to managing relationships is key in encouraging constructive working relationships. This is not to suggest that everybody within a team should be friends, however – this is not realistic and should not be the ultimate aim. Personality issues aside, it is important that teams work through behaviours which are acceptable to everyone.

As Gorman's model also suggests it is important to develop *processes* that enable effective teamworking. Many of these issues have already been covered in depth in earlier chapters so we will not reproduce these discussions here. The final fundamental element of the model (which is interlinked with the other elements) is *culture*. Perceptions, values, language and status are crucial to the way actions and processes are enacted and performed (as discussed in Chapter 3). We expand on this discussion further within the dimensions of the effective partnership working inventory that follows (culture is also explored in depth in the companion text in this series, *Managing and leading in inter-agency settings*, by Edward Peck and Helen Dickinson).

The effective partnership working inventory

The effective partnership working inventory (West and Markiewicz, 2006) aims to measure seven dimensions which are known from research to be critical to the development of effective partnership working – both in multidisciplinary and multiagency teams (illustrated in Figure 4.2). These seven dimensions are further developed in Box 4.1, which gives a list of bullet points illustrating how a partnership

Figure 4.2: Seven dimensions of effective partnership working

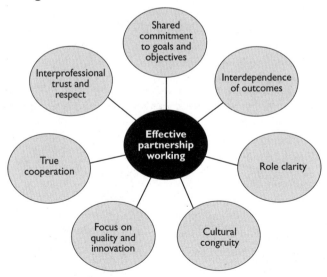

Source: West and Markiewicz (2006)

might check their degree of effectiveness against each of these different competencies. Partnerships might use this inventory to assess which domains they are operating effectively within and which need further development. As this expanded list suggests, teams may need to complete multiple versions of this inventory in respect of the different links they have in terms of the team itself, its own organisation(s) and wider partners. Readers of this book might wish to use this inventory to highlight any areas in which their team needs to develop and then use the tools offered in this chapter to aid this process.

Box 4.1: The dimensions of effective partnership working expanded

Shared commitment to goals and objectives
All partnership members:

- Are clear about their own home team and organisation's goals
- Are clear about the partnership's goals
- Believe that the goals of the partnership are valuable
- Enter into the partnership willingly

Interdependence of outcomes
All partnership members believe:

- Their home team's, organisation's and partnership's goals are interdependent
- Innovation is required to achieve these goals
- The skills and experience brought to the partnership by all the different partners are essential to success

Role clarity
All partnership members:

- Understand their own and each other's role within the partnership

---

- Ensure that power and status relationships are agreed and described
- Work constructively to resolve conflicts which may arise about status or role

Cultural congruity
All partnership members:

- Understand differences between cultures across home teams or across organisational cultures
- Spend time to develop effective processes for working together
- Regularly review working and interpersonal relationships

Focus on quality and innovation
All partnership members:

- Demonstrate a concern for quality which is focused on the aims of the partnership
- Encourage positive challenging and regular constructive debate about working practices
- Share learning from errors or mistakes
- Provide practical support for innovation in working practices

True cooperation
All partnership members:

- Define the requirements for effective partnership working
- Design integrated policies and working practices
- Provide training for partnership working at all levels of the partnership
- Ensure effective communication processes exist and are managed effectively

Interprofessional trust and respect
In relation to other professional groups within the partnership, all individuals:

- Understand the professional roles of each group
- Understand the different ways of working traditionally adopted by each group
- Use positive language to describe the role and contribution of others
- Provide constructive feedback to colleagues from all professional groups

Source: West and Markiewicz (2006)

These seven dimensions shape the rest of this chapter. Each dimension is taken individually and is enhanced by frameworks, tools and models designed to help teams work with and further understand these dimensions in order to enhance effectiveness.

Shared commitment to goals and objectives

As previously suggested, team members need to perceive the team's task to be relevant to the overall aims of the organisation or to a specific part of the organisation to which they can relate. Individuals are motivated by being part of and contributing to a 'bigger cause', and teams that have a clear relationship with the organisation's goals are far less likely to become competitive with other teams. The ability to clearly link the aims and objectives of each team to those of the organisation is essential if synergy of outcomes and clear lines of accountability are to be achieved. The framework presented in Table 4.1, developed by Aston OD (2007), encourages teams to consider how their work links to the wider organisational objectives and to highlight areas in need of improvement.

Of course, the reality is that organisational objectives are not always understood by individuals and teams working at all levels of the organisation. Sometimes this is because of the way organisational

—

Table 4.1: Increasing task relevance

What does the team need to do to improve its understanding of organisational objectives?	Who will the team go to for support?	Specific questions or areas of uncertainty:	Completion date:	Coordinating team member:
What does the team need to do to clarify team objectives and clarify the link between team and organisational objectives?	Who will the team go to for support?	Who do we need to ensure understands our team's contribution to organisational aims?	Completion date:	Coordinating team member:
What will the team stop doing, because this activity is no longer relevant to the organisation's aims or objectives?	Who do we need to tell?	What are our reasons?	Completion date:	Coordinating team member:
What should the organisation add to its aims and objectives?	Who will the team need to influence?	What is our case – what internal or external drivers does this relate to?	Completion date:	Coordinating team member:
What will the team do to increase the contribution it is making to the achievement of organisational aims or objectives?	Whose agreement will the team need?	What actions need to be taken by the team?	Completion date:	Coordinating team member:

Source: Aston OD (2007)

85

Table 4.2: Linking team and organisational objectives

List the organisation's aims or objectives here:

Organisation's aim or objectives	Contributing team's objectives

List the team's objectives here:

	Team's objectives
1	
2	
3	
4	
5	
6	
7	
8	

Show which of your team's objectives contribute to each of the organisation's aims or objectives, by writing the number of the team objective in the second column of the top chart. Each team objective may contribute to only one or to several organisational aims or objectives.

Source: Aston OD (2007)

objectives and expectations of teams have been communicated (or not), and often teams find it hard to relate their day-to-day work to the wider organisation, which can seem remote. But teams need organisations and organisations certainly need teams, and the framework in Table 4.2 is a way of clarifying exactly how team objectives link to and reflect those of the organisation. This is a seemingly simple tool, but often these steps are not considered as teams go straight into action, causing real potential for a lack of synergy and conflict around the work of the team.

To conclude this section it is perhaps helpful to consider the usefulness of a team vision. Effective team visions are valuable – they provide clarity to the team's identity both within and outside the team; provide motivation to team members; enable work to be prioritised; and provide a focus for the development of effective team objectives. However, team vision statements are only effective if they are developed by the team and if they evolve with the team as it develops. It is therefore important to take time out occasionally to review the relevance of the team vision, especially in times of significant change when the team vision can provide either reassurance about the continuing focus of the team's work in the context of structural change, or an energising focus to support a positive view of change. In interprofessional and multidisciplinary teams, the development of a vision statement also provides the opportunity to develop deeper understanding of cultural traditions, differences in language patterns and styles of working.

Interdependence of outcomes

The team's task should require team members to work interdependently. Teams are most useful where the task demands a range of skills that are held by, or best developed by, a number of different individuals. If the team task is designed in such a way that individuals with differing skills and experience do not have the opportunity to work closely together, communicating regularly, sharing information and debating decisions about the best way to do the job, then the team will not realise the opportunities for innovation that are inherent in teamworking. Team location can affect the ability of team members to work interdependently and therefore those teams that are dispersed geographically will need to ensure that communication processes are geared to enabling the best possible interaction of individuals (Cameron and Lart, 2003). A key enabling element of interdependence is trust, which is why interdependence is often difficult to develop and maintain. Trust is hard won and easily lost, and in modern organisations where accountability is often individually attributed, some individuals may feel that trusting others and working truly interdependently is a risky business. There are also a range of tools and approaches that can be useful in surfacing all the outcomes which a team and organisation are working towards. The evaluation text in this series by Helen Dickinson (*Evaluating outcomes in health and social care*) gives an overview of some of these techniques and readers interested in this issue may wish to consult this text.

Role clarity

The importance of role clarity cannot be underestimated. Examples in this book have shown that confusion over role can lead to poor relationships, stress, negative impact on service users and possible duplication of work. This section initially focuses on general roles but then goes on to highlight a model that may be especially useful for team leaders. Effective interprofessional teamworking is above all about producing synergy, where the combined effect of all professional contributions exceeds the sum of the potential individual effects. Synergy may come from:

Understanding – roles, skills, knowledge, expertise, ambitions
Respecting – beliefs, working style
Valuing – contributions, ideas, difference

The following exercise (Table 4.3) provides a structure within which team members can review their individual understanding of others' knowledge, skills and job roles. It also provides a format for pooling

Table 4.3: The role clarity review grid

Please place a cross in the column that best represents your view

Names of individuals or professional groups	How much do you know about this individual or group's job content?				How much do you know about this individual or group's knowledge, skills and ways of working?					How well does this individual or group use your knowledge and skills?			
	Nothing	Very little	A fair amount	A great deal	Nothing	Very little	A fair amount	A great deal	Very poorly	To a limited extent	Well	Very well

Source: Aston OD (2007)

and comparing understanding in order to identify areas in which there is a need for more clarity. In order to use this approach:

- Create a list of team members or, if there are more than 10 team members, the names of different professional groups within your team.
- Write the names of team members or professional groups in the first column of the role clarity review grid (Table 4.3).
- Ask all team members to complete the review grid.
- When all team members have completed the review grid use the information provided to identify areas in which greater clarity is required and to design ways in which this can be achieved.

Leading teams

Team leadership is proposed to be a critical dimension of effective teams. Although leadership is covered in great depth in another book in this series (Peck and Dickinson, 2008), given this proposed importance we provide a model of leadership which may be helpful to team leaders, in addition to Kogler Hill's model (2004) which was illustrated earlier in Chapter 2 (see Figure 2.2). Hackman's (2002) model of the functions of a team leader is based on studies across a wide diversity of teams and their leaders, including sports, business and flight teams (Box 4.2). This model of leadership is about working with individuals to develop a shared accountability for the quality of service the team provides. The focus of this model sees the leader coaching and supporting the team to achieve. What is fundamental is that team leaders working in this way take time to clarify their role with the rest of the team. If roles, responsibilities and expectations are not clear, there is real potential for conflict to arise. This model may be unfamiliar to some team members who are used to (and may even prefer) more traditional models of leadership (where power is held and exercised by virtue of hierarchical position), and it may take time for them to come to understand the power of leadership being enacted in this way. Finally, it is pertinent to raise the issue of support for team leaders who are often facing difficult challenges and problems. If they really are to coach and facilitate it is essential they have the

—

confidence to do so, which means organisations must invest and make this support accessible.

Box 4.2: The functions of a team leader

Create favourable performance conditions for the team

- Ensure there is a well-defined task
- Ensure the team has the necessary organisational resources and clear boundaries
- Use resources, authority and influence to create a good working environment

Build and maintain the team as a performing unit

- Ensure the team has the right skill mix to meet service needs
- Create processes to facilitate the team to perform effectively

Coach and support the team

- Support and work with individuals and the team as a collective whole
- Champion team and individual learning and development
- Pay attention to relationships and processes which impact on performance

Source: Hackman (2002)

Cultural congruity

Describing culture has been described as a bit like nailing jelly to a wall. Culture is hard to get hold of (or define) and articulate, but people tacitly know what is meant by this term. Ouchi and Johnson (1978) describe culture as 'the way we do things around here', suggesting it is representative of a habitual, traditional way of thinking, being and feeling. Morgan (1986) describes culture as 'the pattern of interaction, the language that is used, the images and themes explored in conversation, and the various rituals of daily routine'. As Schein (1985) suggests, culture is manifested at many different levels, in thoughts and language as well as material artefacts. The result of this is a paradoxical situation where culture is hard to describe, but is fundamental for effective teamworking. *Managing and leading in inter-agency settings*, by Edward Peck and Helen Dickinson (in this series), gives very detailed consideration of culture and its implications in a partnership setting, so we do not repeat these discussions here. However, Table 4.4 sets out a framework that has been developed by Aston OD for analysing interprofessional culture in teams. It has been extensively used to assess interagency work between public and private sectors and is offered here as a framework that can be adapted to suit specific working partnerships and teams.

Focus on quality and innovation

Much is written in the literature about the ability of effective teams to be creative and innovative and it is perhaps important to distinguish between creativity and innovation and to emphasise their relationships with improving services. Creativity is not necessarily about completely new ideas, which can seem a daunting, unobtainable ideal. Instead, 'creativity is the connecting and rearranging of knowledge – in the minds of people who will allow them to think flexibly – to generate new, often surprising ideas that others judge to be useful' (Plsek, 1997, p 27). *Creativity* is therefore the new idea and *innovation* is the implementing of the idea or way of working in order to *improve* service delivery. This section highlights a few models and tools to facilitate the innovation process, but it is important first of all to focus on the outcomes of implementing new ideas.

It should be noted that not all changes or innovations are improvements – some may potentially have negative impacts. Evaluation should be built into all improvement processes to measure the impact of the improvement and to stop it if it is not doing what was hoped. However, evaluation is often forgotten – or overlooked

Table 4.4: Interprofessional culture review

The following sets of statements represent 'poles' of ways in which groups can work. Please shade in a square to show where you would place your professional group on each cultural dimension.

Relationship to the environment					
Our professional group tends to believe it is not as valuable as other groups in the organisation or partnership					Our professional group believes that its contribution is more important than most others to the achievement of the organisation's goals
Most staff in our professional group would regard themselves as members of the organisation first and members of their profession second					Most staff in our professional group would regard themselves as members of their profession first and members of the organisation second
The nature of human activity					
In our professional group we value competitive behaviour and reward those who are proactive and go all out to win					In our professional group we value most those people who create harmony and are willing to go with the flow
In our profession staff tend to be promoted on the basis of individual achievement in a specialist field					In our profession staff tend to be promoted on the basis of their ability to coordinate and integrate the work of others
Testing reality					
In our professional group we need hard evidence and a good deal of data before we move forward with any major activity					In our professional group we often take decisions without a great deal of data, relying more on the gut feel of key individuals
Our profession is often regarded as conservative and cautious in its approach					Our profession is generally seen to be quick to react to changes in the external environment
Time focus and formality					
Staff in our profession tend to talk a lot about our past victories and the ways in which we have traditionally worked					Staff in our profession tend to talk a great deal about the future and the ways in which it will be different from the past
In our professional group major decisions take a great deal of time and are discussed at length by numerous groups of people					Our professional group often surprises partners and colleagues by our speed of decision taking and rapid progress to action

(continued)

Table 4.4: Interprofessional culture review (continued)

The nature of human nature						
In our professional group we expect people to be up to speed when they join us and contribute immediately						In our professional group we expect people to need time to 'settle in' before they can make a major contribution
People in our group often refer to others as 'brilliant' or 'useless' at their job						People in our group tend to assume everyone is capable of being good at their job
Work relationships						
In our profession we enjoy our competitive environment and people are rewarded for the results they individually contribute						In our profession we reward people as a group and expect all individuals to be effective team workers
We have a very hierarchical structure						We make huge efforts to include everyone in decision making
Homogeneity versus diversity						
Historically our working groups have been pretty homogeneous – we tend to come from the same professional background and be very similar in other ways too						Historically our working groups have been very diverse, employees come from many professional backgrounds and there is a great deal of individual difference between staff members
Most of the jobs in our profession are carried out in similar ways						Jobs within our profession require a variety of ways of working

Source: Aston OD (2007)

within busy environments – with the result that many changes that are not improvements continue. The model in Figure 4.3 is known as the Plan, Do, Study and Act (PDSA) model and is recognised as a model for improvement that helps a team to set aims, targets and measures, and introduces a way of testing ideas before implementing them (Langley et al, 1996). There are two stages to successfully using the model. The first is to consider three questions:

1. What are we trying to accomplish?
2. How will we know that change is an improvement?
3. What changes can we make that will result in improvement?

Then plan the improvement, try it out, observe the results and, importantly, act on the learning.

Figure 4.3: The PDSA cycle

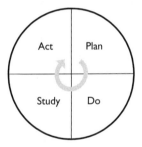

Having identified a recognised process for the implementation of ideas it seems important to highlight some of the principles that underpin tools and exercises associated with creative thinking. The model in Figure 4.4 illustrates the principles of creative thinking as suggested by Plsek (1997). Most of the tools which seek to assist these processes start by focusing on an area which needs improving and then trying to escape from current ways of seeing the issue in order to move thinking to a different place. Such models try to get beyond current ways of conceptualising and responding to issues as these often set

Figure 4.4: Principles of creative thinking

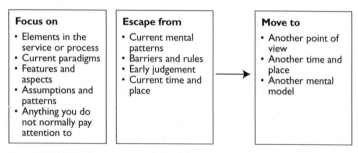

Focus on	Escape from	Move to
• Elements in the service or process • Current paradigms • Features and aspects • Assumptions and patterns • Anything you do not normally pay attention to	• Current mental patterns • Barriers and rules • Early judgement • Current time and place	• Another point of view • Another time and place • Another mental model

Source: Plsek (1997)

the parameters of what it 'thinkable' within that context. By focusing on what it is that you are aiming to achieve it is often easier to come up with more innovative ideas than if you start from the basis of what currently happens. As an example, an integrated children's team, which one of the authors worked with, reported consistent difficulties in accessing respite services. This was often brought up as a major obstacle for the team, with seemingly no obvious way to overcome this difficulty due to a lack of respite resources in the locality. However, once the team started to think about what it was they were actually trying to achieve (that is, outcomes for children and families, rather than services), they produced a list of innovative ways in which they could meet these needs (for example, through direct payments), which did not involve accessing more respite services.

Creativity will remain an idealised concept unless organisations and managers create conditions where it can truly flourish. People need time and space in order to be able to think differently, which usually has resource implications (either in terms of time or money). One tool that can be used to aid practical, creative thinking is de Bono's (1985) 'thinking hats' technique (Figure 4.5). The thinking hats tool is made up of six different hats that represent different ways of thinking about an issue. Teams should use this tool to consider 'one hat' at a time and think through the implications of this factor. In other words, entire teams (or small groups) systematically think through an issue from a variety of different perspectives. When discussing issues one viewpoint

—

Figure 4.5: Edward de Bono's six thinking hats

White hat
Information

- Information we know
- Information we would like to know
- Information we need
- Information that is missing
- How are we going to get that information
- Includes hard facts to doubtful information

Red hat
Feelings, intuition, emotions

- Permission to express feelings
- No need to justify
- Represents feeling right now
- Keep it short
- A key ingredient in decision making

Black hat
Logical negative

- The pessimistic view
- Reasons must be given
- Points out thinking that does not fit the facts, experience, regulations, strategy, values
- Points out potential problems
- The most useful hat

Yellow hat
Logical positive

- The optimistic view
- Reasons must be given
- Needs more effort than the black hat
- Looks for the concept behind the idea

Green hat
New ideas, possibilities

- Creative thinking
- Seeking alternatives and possibilities
- Removing faults
- Doesn't have to be logical
- Generates new concepts

Blue hat
Managing the thinking

- 'Control' hat
- Organises the thinking
- Sets the focus and agenda
- Summarises and concludes
- Ensures that the rules are observed

will often have a tendency to dominate, but using this technique means that emotions, hard facts and the positives and negatives associated with an issue are all given a hearing. Often we do not recognise that we are thinking about a problem in a particular way. If we do not like something or are negative about an issue we may not recognise that we are conceptualising this in a pessimistic manner. By hearing different viewpoints, or thinking about an issue from a different perspective, this should become apparent. It can often be a useful exercise to try and think about such an issue with a 'yellow hat' and think through all the potential positives that are associated with it. Similarly, when we have a good idea it is easy to get carried away. It may be useful in these situations to put on the 'black hat' and seriously think through any potential negatives that might be associated with this idea.

Using the de Bono tool is one way of hearing a range of voices and issues that may otherwise be subsumed in discussions around complex issues. However, simply deciding on the course of action for the future is not quite the end of the process. Without managers giving sufficient freedom to individuals and teams to make decisions over an issue, they can do all the creative thinking they want but will not be able to act on it. This is illustrative of the way in which many of the factors in the effective partnership working inventory are interlinked.

True cooperation

True cooperation is about co-processing and necessitating interaction around interdependent processes; it is not about separate parallel worlds. Therefore, for real cooperation to exist individuals need to be very clear about who they are cooperating with, why and how, and decision making and communication processes are key. Communication has been mentioned frequently throughout this book, but it is a very real obstacle that many teams encounter problems with. One model that is being increasingly used by teams in a variety of care environments to better communicate in order to improve safety is the SBAR model:

- *Situation:* a concise statement of the problem
- *Background:* pertinent and brief information related to the situation

- *Assessment:* analysis and consideration of options
- *Recommendation:* action/recommendations

Using this approach gives a predictable structure to communication (see Box 4.3). This has been standard procedure within the aviation industry but is less widely used throughout health and social care (although some areas of clinical medicine have started to adopt this approach at the start of shifts, for example). Haig et al (2006) demonstrate how this tool has been successfully used in teams in North America and Australia to improve communication by structuring conversations within and across teams.

Box 4.3: Using the SBAR approach

Outlining *Situation* should pick up any potential difficulties with different professional approaches to language and narrative. Individuals should clearly and briefly state the problem in a way that others understand. The information shared at this stage should cover exactly what the problem is. For example, "Dr Khan, I'm calling about Mrs Weston, who is experiencing increased anxiety".

The *Background* provides information that is succinct, pertinent and factual. What were the circumstances leading up to this problem? "She is a 74-year-old woman who is receiving medication for anxiety, but is getting much worse."

With *Assessment* the conversation moves on to an analysis of the current situation and leads to what you think the problem is. "She is constantly 'phoning about problems and she has not left the house for two weeks."

The conversation ends on *Recommendation* where specific actions are outlined and agreed on clearly. This is the area that often fails in communication processes, as different parties are not clear about the action and priority of the next steps. "I need you to see her today at your out-patient clinic. She needs her medication reviewing and referral to a psychologist."

Source: Based on Leonard et al (2004)

The SBAR model is based on the principles of the assertion cycle (Figure 4.6). One of the difficulties of communication is that it is influenced by social processes. Individuals may feel constrained by issues of hierarchy or power and unable to state a problem and secure an answer. Often people speak indirectly and hint at the existence of a problem and hope that colleagues pick up on this. But there are clearly quite large risk implications here. The assertion cycle states a problem politely and persistently until they get an answer. If all members of a team are used to using this approach then if an individual states "I need to see you now", their colleague knows that this cannot wait. Although this clearly has applications within critical care contexts, it is equally applicable to primary care and community settings.

Figure 4.6: The assertion cycle

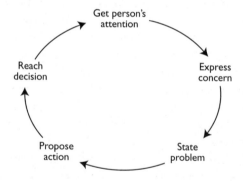

Interprofessional trust and respect

The importance of trust and respect has been highlighted throughout this book and it is undoubtedly a major issue for many individuals working in teams. As we have argued, it takes time for trust to develop, but organisations engaged in a whirlwind of change, often with the goal of improving services, sometimes forget this. Without trust people will not take risks and without risks people will not undertake to do things differently. The model described by Lencioni (2002) (Figure 4.7)

Figure 4.7: The five dysfunctions of a team

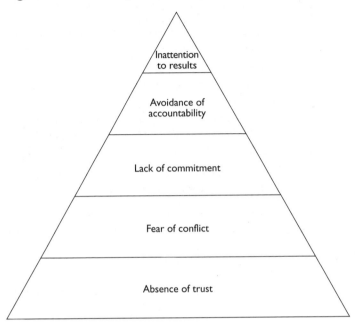

Source: Lencioni (2002, p 188)

tries to get to grips with the issue of why so many teams struggle. It is presented as a hierarchy with interdependencies between each level. Absence of trust is the foundation that leads to the potential for more dysfunction to develop if it is not present, respected and nurtured. The five dysfunctions are:

- *Absence of trust:* this factor relates not just to individuals trusting each other but also reluctance to be seen as vulnerable. If individuals are unable (or feel unable) to be open with one another about their weaknesses and mistakes then it is impossible to build a foundation for trust to develop. This also returns to an earlier message in the book, that people need to trust each other in order to take risks and to improve services through innovation. Lack of stability is often the reason that people struggle to develop trusting relationships with each other as they do not know each other and so cannot sufficiently predict what the future actions of their partners will be.

- *Fear of conflict:* this is at the heart of many of the problems in dysfunctional teams. People are afraid to, or do not know how to, manage conflict and it is therefore often left to fester and grow into something destructive that has a major impact on a range of people. Conflict is often seen negatively rather than as difference of opinion between two parties that needs working through. Avoiding conflict may mean that there is not a culture of challenge and passionate debate in teams (elements that are positively associated with safety). Investment in conflict resolution skills for staff working at all levels of systems should be a major priority for all organisations in health and social care.

- *Lack of commitment:* for Lencioni, this is about individuals not committing to decisions and then subsequently undermining decisions the team has made.

- *Avoidance of accountability:* this is the reluctance to hold people to account for their practice, behaviours and actions that might be counterproductive to the effectiveness of the team.

- *Inattention to results:* this occurs when people put their individual needs, wishes and interests above the collective goals of the team.

As a working tool it is suggested that people are familiar with the five stages of the model and the meaning and interpretation of each dysfunction. They then need to analyse the team (either alone or with the team) to explore perceptions, reality and feelings about each dimension and then, importantly, to decide on any action that needs to be taken.

Overall, this chapter has sought to provide an overview of some key frameworks, models and tools that may help to develop and enhance understanding of effective teamworking. Central to this process is the need to take time to reflect on what the issues really are (the what) and then to further reflect on the best way forward (the how and the who). Indeed, this is a key message of this entire book, that partnerships need to be clear about what they are trying to achieve and use these aims to inform the structure and processes of subsequent relationships. All too often teams (understandably) get wrapped up with the way in which things currently do or do not work, without looking above the immediate context and seeing what could be. As suggested early on in Chapter 1, real teams have a clear focus on what it is they are trying to achieve by working together. By bearing these aims in mind and employing some of the frameworks and models outlined in this chapter, teams should be able to work together more effectively.

Reflective exercises

1. Create a representation of the adapted Gorman model (Figure 4.1). Where are the strengths and areas that need developing in your team?

2. Consider another team or organisation that you are working in partnership with and reflect on the dimensions of the effective partnership working inventory (Figure 4.2 and Box 4.1).

3. Think about the frameworks of leadership suggested in this chapter (Box 4.2). What do you do well and what do you need to develop? What would your team members say?

4. Consider your approach to a recent change in service. How well did the process reflect the stages of the Plan, Do, Study and Act model (Figure 4.3)?

5. Think about a decision you have to take, or an issue that you are working on and apply de Bono's thinking hats (Figure 4.5). Start with the facts (white hat) and work through the remaining colours.

6. Think about recent team meetings. How well are people able to assert their views? Use the stages in the assertion model (Figure 4.6) to help your thinking.

7. Think about Lencioni's model of a dysfunctional team (Figure 4.7). What does your team do well, and not so well?

Further reading and resources

References relating to key texts underpinning the chapter can be found in the final References section at the end of the book. In addition:

- ITMA is an integrated team monitoring and assessment tool that is freely available for integrated teams in order to provide a relatively simple and cost-effective way of assessing the effectiveness of teamworking. It enables a rapid appraisal of the 'health' of a team and identifies areas of difficulty covering both internal functioning and external factors, thereby enabling a focus on remedial action commensurate with the significance of the problems: www.integratedcarenetwork.gov.uk/_library/Resources/ICN/publications/ITMA_May_Launch_Version.doc

- Accessible information about coaching and mentoring may be found at The Coaching and Mentoring Network. This site is primarily aimed at coaches and people looking for coaches, but has a good resource centre which is freely available and contains full text articles, case studies and up-to-date news: www.coachingnetwork.org.uk

- The Consortium for Research on Emotional Intelligence in Organisations facilitates the advancement of research and practice relevant to emotional intelligence in organisations. The website contains full text articles, research papers, reports and guidelines: www.eiconsortium.org

- The Chartered Institute of Personnel and Development is the UK's leading professional body for those involved in the management and development of people. Many selected resources, papers and tools are free: www.cipd.co.uk

- Paul Plsek's site DirectedCreativity™ has a wealth of tools and information around the issue of creativity: www.directedcreativity.com

5

Recommendations for policy and practice

Ultimately, the evidence, questions, summaries, learning and frameworks set out in this book lead us to make a series of practical recommendations and potential warnings, both for policy and for practice.

For policy makers:

- There is a need to consider the implications for existing teams and services when they exhort new teams or style of working. Creating new teams in any area will affect existing teams, their working practices and relationships, and may hinder the development of practice as people struggle to differentiate roles and boundaries.

- Measures of teams in organisations are sometimes only built around their existence, not around their effectiveness; this perhaps adds to cynicism around rhetoric, as opposed to commitment, to teamworking.

- Although teamworking may be helpful in a number of ways, it is not a default position that will solve all difficulties. Teams need real tasks and a real need to work together in order to be effective. Simply ordering more of certain types of teams will not overcome the difficulties which health and social care communities face.

- There is a real imperative for joined-up policies. For example, there has been a great deal of rhetoric around teamworking, but Agenda for Change is geared around and reinforces individual reward. Furthermore, policies need interdependent priorities. For example, the priorities for a PCT chief executive may be different to a prison governor, but with PCTs now accountable for the provision of healthcare needs there has to be common ground. Prison service orders and Department of Health guidance need to have synergy; real partnerships are about a common interest in each other achieving goals.

- National policy needs to send out stronger messages about how organisations need to make investments in enhancing and sustaining teamworking, rather than just one-off training.

- There is a real need to have some stability in the system. Improvement in services is about doing something differently. To do this, people need to take risks and they will not feel safe to do so until there is a climate of mutual trust and respect, which takes time to develop.

- There is an increasing tendency within commissioning to design specific care pathways (that is, for certain conditions or client groups), rather than commissioning particular professional services (for example, district nursing services). The implication of this is that there will be a greater demand to work across boundaries and for individual professionals to work as teams. World class commissioning should demand that appropriate support and development needs to be made available to support professionals and teamworking in these roles.

For local organisations and frontline services:

- Do not underestimate the power and importance of teamworking. There is a tendency in health and social care settings not to prioritise team development, as care inputs are seen as more immediately important. However, team development and teamworking do have real implications for the quality of services delivered, particularly within interagency settings. At the same time people need to be encouraged to think about whether the task in hand really needs a team – there is a need for teams to tackle real issues as conflict is draining and impacts on everyone.

- Teams really do need time to be teams. Just putting everyone together and expecting them to work effectively without ever being able to meet, debate and explore will not work. Evidence is very clear about the importance of creating conditions to develop reflexivity and the subsequent relationship to improved innovation and quality of services. Overt organisational commitment to this is crucial. We need clear messages from leaders in organisations that time for teams is valuable and supported.

- New ways of working and the associated new design of facilities can mean that traditional ways of meeting are getting harder. If teams are to be effective they need to be able to meet, and they need somewhere to do so!

- If there are to be changes around teamworking or integration, leaders must take time to find out about how people are currently working. Much more partnership and teamworking is taking place than is recognised. The work of practitioners and existing teams needs to be valued.

- The increasing development towards the commissioning of care pathways as opposed to the commissioning of professional services will see the need to work across boundaries and teamworking increase. As a result, the key issues and frameworks in this book will become even more important over time.

- Research tells us that middle managers are under the most stress and there are often no easy answers to many of the complex problems and issues that they are facing. However, investment in development in the form of mentoring, coaching and learning sets may provide valuable returns.

So, finally, there really are no great secrets about teamworking, but different knowledge levels, skills, intuition and experiences make it a contested arena. It is not a panacea for all situations, but an area that needs real commitment, investment and curiosity. The conditions for the nurturing of teams are crucial. Inhospitable conditions will mean that they wither and fail to grow. Some commitment to create the right conditions will see some growth. But real commitment to creating the right environment will likely see teams flourish, unleashing potential and energy that will take them in often surprising directions in their quest to develop innovative services and care (see Figure 5.1).

Figure 5.1: Nurturing the effectiveness of teams

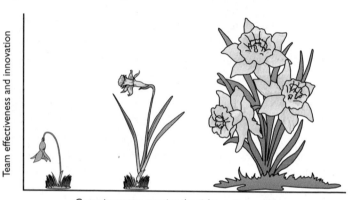

Team effectiveness and innovation

Commitment to creating the right environment

References

6, P., Glasby, J. and Lester, H. (2007) 'Incremental change without policy learning: explaining information rejection in English mental health services', *Journal of Comparative Policy Analysis*, vol 9, pp 21-46.

6, P., Leat, D., Seltzer, K. and Stoker, G. (2002) *Towards holistic governance: The new reform agenda*, New York, NY: Palgrave.

Adair, J. (1986) *Effective team building*, London: Gower.

Adair, J. (1997) *Decision making and problem solving*, Channel Isles: The Guernsey Press.

Allen, N. and Hecht, T. (2004) 'The "romance" of teams: toward an understanding of its psychological underpinnings and implications', *Journal of Occupational and Organizational Psychology*, vol 77, pp 439-61.

Allison, G. and Zelikow, P. (1999) *Essence of decision: Explaining the Cuban missile crisis*, Harlow: Longman.

Anning, A. and Edwards, A. (1999) *Promoting children's learning from birth to five: Developing the new Early Years professional*, Buckingham: Open University Press.

Appelbaum, E. and Batt, R. (1994) *The new American workplace*, Ithaca, NY: ILR Press.

Argyris, C. and Schön, D. (1978) *Organizational learning: A theory of action perspective*, Reading, MA: Addison Wesley.

Aston OD (Organisation Development) (2007) 'The Aston team performance toolkit' (available from www.astonod.com).

Audit Commission (1992) *Homeward bound: A new course for community health*, London: HMSO.

Baggott, R. (2000) *Public health: Policy and politics*, Basingstoke: Macmillan Press Ltd.

Balloch, S. and Taylor, M. (2001) *Partnership working: Policy and practice*, Bristol: The Policy Press.

Barr, H., Koppel, I., Reeves, S., Hammick, M. and Freeth, D. (2005) *Effective interprofessional education: Argument, assumption and evidence*, Oxford: Blackwell Publishing.

Barrett, G., Sellman, D. and Thomas, J. (eds) (2005) *Interprofessional working in health and social care: Professional perspectives*, Basingstoke: Palgrave.

BBC (British Broadcasting Corporation) (2003) 'Trusts to take over child care', 28 January (www.bbc.co.uk, accessed 20/04/2007).

BBC (2005) '"Home alone" deaths for thousands, 29 December (www.bbc.co.uk, accessed 16/02/2007).

Belbin, M. (2000) *Beyond the team*, Oxford: Butterworth-Heinemann.

Bevan, H. (2006) 'On email-tyranny', *Health Services Journal*, 12 January, p 23.

BMA (British Medical Association) (1974) *Primary health care teams*, London: BMA.

Borrill, C., West, M., Carter, M. and Dawson, J. (2003) *The relationship between staff satisfaction and patient satisfaction*, Research Paper, Aston: Aston Business School.

Borrill, C., Carletta, J., Carter, A., Dawson, J., Garrod, S., Rees, A., Richards, A., Shapiro, D. and West, M. (2001) *The effectiveness of health care teams in the National Health Service*, Aston: Aston Centre for Health Service Organization Research.

Bostock, L., Bairstow, S., Fish, S. and Macleod, F. (2005) *Managing risk and minimising mistakes to services for children and families*, London: Social Care Institute for Excellence.

British Medical Journal (2004) 'Ombudsman', *British Medical Journal*, vol 328, p 10.

Brown, L., Tucker, C. and Domokos, T. (2003) 'Evaluating the impact of integrated health and social care teams on older people living in the community', *Health and Social Care in the Community*, vol 11, pp 85-94.

Burns, L.R. and Pauly, M.V. (2002) 'Integrated delivery networks: a detour on the road to integrated health?', *Business of Health Care*, vol 21, pp 126-43.

Burstow, P. (2005) *Dying alone: Assessing isolation, loneliness and poverty* (www.paulburstow.org.uk).

Cameron, A. and Lart, R. (2003) 'Factors promoting and obstacles hindering joint working: a systematic review of the research evidence', *Journal of Integrated Care*, vol 11, issue 2, pp 9-17.

Carpenter, J. and Barnes, D. (2001) 'Integrating health and social welfare services', in G. Thornicroft and G. Szmukler (eds) *Community psychiatry*, Oxford: Oxford University Press.

Carpenter, J. and Dickinson, H. (2008) *Interprofessional education and training*, Bristol: The Policy Press.

Clegg, S. (2005) *Managing and organisations: An introduction to theory and practice*, London: Sage Publications.

Clutterbuck, D. (2007) *Coaching the team at work*, London: Nicholas Brealey International.

Cohen, S. and Bailey, D. (1997) 'What makes teams work: group effectiveness research from the shop floor to the executive suite', *Journal of Management*, vol 23, pp 239-90.

Cook, G., Gerrish, K. and Clarke, C. (2001) 'Decision-making in teams: issues arising from two UK evaluations', *Journal of Interprofessional Care*, vol 15, pp 141-51.

Cott, C. (1997) 'We decide, you carry it out: a social network analysis of multidisciplinary long-term care teams', *Social Science and Medicine*, vol 45, pp 1411-21.

Craddock, D., Borthwick, A. and McPherson, K. (2006) 'Interprofessional education in health and social care: fashion or informed practice?', *Learning in Health and Social Care*, vol 5, pp 220-42.

Davey, B., Levin, E., Iliffe, S. and Kharicha, K. (2005) 'Integrating health and social care: implications for joint working and community care outcomes for older people', *Journal of Interprofessional Care*, vol 19, pp 22-34.

de Bono, E. (1985) *Six thinking hats*, New York, NY: Little, Brown and Company.

DH (Department of Health) (1998) *Partnership in action: New opportunities for joint working between health and social services*, London: DH.

DH (1999) *Making a difference: Strengthening the nursing, midwifery and health visiting contribution to health and healthcare*, London: DH.

DH (2000) *The NHS Plan: A plan for investment, a plan for reform*, London: The Stationery Office.

DH (2002a) *Liberating the talents: Helping primary care trusts and nurses to deliver the NHS Plan*, London: DH.

DH (2002b) *Community mental health teams*, London: DH.

DH (2002c) *Reform of social work education and training*, London: DH.

DH (2006) *Our health, our care our say: A new direction for community services*, London: The Stationery Office.

Dickinson, H. (2008) *Evaluating outcomes in health and social care*, Bristol: The Policy Press.

Dickinson, H., Peck, E. and Davidson, D. (2007) 'Opportunity seized or missed? A case study of leadership and organizational change in the creation of a care trust', *Journal of Interprofessional Care*, vol 21, no 5, pp 503-13.

Dunn, E., Mills, P., Neily, J., Crittenden, M., Carmack, A. and Baigan, J. (2007) 'Medical team training: applying crew resource management in the Veterans Administration', *The Joint Commission Journal on Quality and Patient Safety*, vol 33, pp 317-24.

Edmonson, A. (1996) 'Learning from mistakes is easier said than done: group and organisational influences on the detection and correction of human error', *Journal of Applied Behavioural Science*, vol 32, pp 5-28.

Edmonson, A. (1999) 'Psychological safety and learning behaviour in work teams', *Administrative Science Quarterly*, vol 44, pp 350-83.

Evetts, J. (1999) 'Professionalisation and professionalism: issues for interprofessional care', *Journal of Interprofessional Care*, vol 13, pp 119-28.

Firth-Cozens, J. (2001) 'Cultures for improving patient safety through learning', *Quality and Safety in Health Care*, vol 10, pp 26-31.

Freeth, D., Hammick, M., Koppel, I., Reeves, S. and Barr, H. (2002) *A critical review of evaluations of interprofessional education*, London: CAIPE.

Gair, G. and Hartley, T. (2001) 'Medical dominance in multidisciplinary teamwork: a case study of discharge decision making in a geriatric assessment unit', *Journal of Nursing Management*, vol 9, pp 3-11.

Glasby, J. and Dickinson, H. (2008) *Partnership working in health and social care*, Bristol: The Policy Press.

Glendinning, C., Powell, M. and Rummery, K. (2002) *Partnerships, New Labour and the governance of welfare*, Bristol: The Policy Press.

GMC (General Medical Council) (2006) *Accountability in multi-disciplinary and multi-agency mental health teams*, London: The Standards and Ethics Committee.

Goodman, S.A. and Svyantek, D.J. (1999) 'Person–organization fit and contextual performance: do shared values matter?', *Journal of Vocational Behavior*, vol 55, pp 254-75.

Gorman, P. (1998) *Managing multidisciplinary teams in the NHS*, London: Kogan Page.

Guzzo, R.A. and Dickson, M.W. (1996) 'Teams in organizations: recent research on performance and effectiveness', *Annual Review of Psychology*, vol 47, pp 307-38.

Hackman, J.R. (1990) *Groups that work (and those that don't): Creating conditions for effective teamwork*, San Francisco, CA: Jossey-Bass.

* Hackman, J.R. (2002) *Leading teams: Setting the stage for great performances*, Boston, MA: Harvard Business School Press.

Haig, K., Sutton, S. and Whittington, J. (2006) 'SBAR: a shared mental model to influence communication between clinicians', *Journal on Quality and Patient Safety*, vol 32, pp 167-75.

Hamman, W. (2004) 'The complexity of team training: what we have learned from aviation and its applications to medicine', *Quality and Safety in Health Care*, vol 13, pp 72-9.

Hastings, A. (1996) 'Unravelling the process of "partnership" in urban regeneration policy', *Urban Studies*, vol 33, no 2, pp 253-68.

Health and Social Care Information Service (2006) 'Data on written complaints in the NHS 2005/06' (www.ic.nhs.uk/, accessed 14/09/2007).

Healthcare Commission (2004) *2003 NHS staff survey*, London: Healthcare Commission.

Healthcare Commission/CSCI (Commission for Social Care Inspection) (2006) *Joint investigation into the provision of services for people with learning disabilities at Cornwall Partnership NHS Trust*, London: Healthcare Commission.

Hébert, R., Tourigny, A. and Gagnon, M. (2005) *Integrated service delivery to ensure persons' functional autonomy*, Québec: EDISEM.

Hodges, S.P. and Hernandez, M. (1999) 'How organizational culture influences outcome information utilization', *Evaluation and Program Planning*, vol 22, pp 183-97.

Home Office (2002) *Prison statistics for England and Wales*, London: The Stationery Office.

Home Office (2006) *Crime in England and Wales 2005/06*, London: Home Office.

Hudson, B. (2000) 'Inter-agency collaboration: a sceptical view', in A. Brechin, H. Brown and M. Eby (eds) *Critical practice in health and social care*, Milton Keynes: Open University Press.

Hudson, B. (2002) 'Interprofessionality in health and social care: the Achilles' heal of partnership?', *Journal of Interprofessional Care*, vol 16, pp 7-17.

Hunter, D.L. (1996) 'The changing roles of health personnel in health and health care management', *Social Science and Medicine*, vol 43, pp 799-808.

Ingram, H. and Desombre, T. (1999) 'Teamwork in health care: lessons from the literature and from good practice around the world', *Journal of Management in Medicine*, vol 13, pp 51-8.

Irvine, R., Kerridge, I., McPhee, J. and Freeman, S. (2002) 'Interprofessionalism and ethics: consensus or clash of cultures?', *Journal of Interprofessional Care*, vol 16, pp 199-210.

Jackson, G., Gater, R., Goldberg, D., Tantam, D., Loftus, L. and Taylor, H. (1993) 'A new community mental health team based in primary care: a description of the service and its effect on service use in the first year', *British Journal of Psychiatry*, vol 162, pp 375-84.

Jackson, S.E., Brett, J., Sessa, V., Cooper, D., Julin, J. and Peyronnin, K. (1991) 'Some differences make a difference: individual dissimilarity and group heterogeneity as correlates of recruitment, promotions, and turnover', *Journal of Applied Psychology*, vol 76, pp 675-89.

Janis, I.L. (1972) *Victims of groupthink*, Boston, MA: Houghton Mifflin Company.

Jelphs, K. (2006) 'Communication: soft skill, hard impact?', *Clinician in Management*, vol 14, pp 33-7.

Johri, M., Béland, F. and Bergman, H. (2003) 'International experiments in integrated care for the elderly: a synthesis of the evidence', *International Journal of Geriatric Psychiatry*, vol 18, pp 222-35.

Jones, R. (2004) 'Bringing health and social care together for older people: Wiltshire's journey from independence to interdependence to integration', *Journal of Integrated Care*, vol 12, pp 27-32.

Jupp, B. (2000) *Working together: Creating a better environment for cross-sector partnerships*, London: Demos.

Kane, R., Illston, L. and Miller, N. (1992) 'Qualitative analysis of the program of all-inclusive care for the elderly (PACE)', *The Gerontologist*, vol 32, pp 771-80.

Katon, W., Von Korff, M. and Lin, E. (1999) 'Stepped collaborative care for primary care patients with persistent symptoms of depression: a randomized trial', *Archives of General Psychiatry*, vol 56, pp 1109-15.

Katzenbach, J. and Smith, D. (1993) *The wisdom of teams*, Boston, MA: Harvard Business School Press.

Klijn, E.-H. and Koppenjan, J.F.M. (2000) 'Public management and policy networks: foundations of a network approach to governance', *Public Management*, vol 2, pp 135-58.

Kodner, D.L. and Kay Kyriacou, C. (2000) 'Fully integrated care for the frail elderly: two American models', *International Journal of Integrated Care*, vol 1.

• Kogler Hill, S. (2004) 'Team leadership', in P. Northouse (ed) *Leadership theory and practice*, London: Sage Publications.

Laming, H. (2003) *The Victoria Climbié Inquiry: Report of an inquiry*, London: The Stationery Office.

* Langley, G., Nolan, K., Nolan, T., Norman, C. and Provost, L. (1996) *The improvement guide: A practical approach to enhancing organisational performance*, San Francisco, CA: Jossey-Bass.

Leape, L. (1994) 'Error in medicine', *The Journal of the American Medical Association*, vol 272, pp 1851-7.

Lencioni, P. (2002) *The five dysfunctions of a team*, San Francisco, CA: Jossey- Bass.

Leonard, M., Graham, S. and Bonacum, D. (2004) 'The human factor: the critical importance of effective teamwork and communication in providing safe care', *Quality and Safety in Health Care*, vol 13, pp 85-90.

Levy, P.F. (2001) 'The Nut Island effect: when good teams go wrong', *Harvard Business Review*, vol 9, pp 51-9.

McCulloch, A. and Parker, C. (2004) 'Inquiries, assertive outreach and compliance: is there a relationship?', in N. Stanley and J. Manthorpe (eds) *The age of inquiry: Learning and blaming in health and social care*, London: Routledge.

McIntyre, R.M. and Salas, E. (1995) 'Measuring and managing for team performance: lessons from complex environments', in R.A. Guzzo and E. Salas (eds) *Team effectiveness and decision making in organizations*, San Francisco, CA: Jossey-Bass.

Macdonald, P. (1990) *Group support technologies*, Report written for the Organizations Planning and Development Division, Office of Human Resource Management, Federal Aviation Administration, US Department of Transportation Systems Centre, Strategic Management Division, Cambridge, MA.

Macy, B. and Izumi, H. (1993) 'Organizational change, design and work innovation: a meta-analysis of 131 North American field studies – 1961-1991,' in W. Passmore and R. Woodman (eds) *Research in organizational change and design*, vol 7, Greenwich, CT: JAI Press.

Martin, V. (2003) *Leading change in health and social care*, London: Routledge.

Mathieson, S. (2006) 'NHS should embrace lean times', *Society Guardian*, 8 June (www.guardian.co.uk/society/2006/jun/08/health. publicservices).

Mehrabian, A. (1972) *Nonverbal communication*, Chicago, IL: Aldine-Atherton. Mickan, S.M. and Rodger, S.A. (2005) 'Effective health care teams: a model of six characteristics developed from shared perceptions', *Journal of Interprofessional Care*, vol 18, pp 358-70.

Miller, C., Freeman, M. and Ross, N. (2001) *Interprofessional practice in health and social care: Challenging the shared learning agenda*, London: Arnold.

Mohrman, S.A., Cohen, S.G. and Mohrman, A.M. (1995) *Designing team-based organizations*, San Francisco, CA: Jossey-Bass.

Morgan, G. (1986) *Images of organization*, London: Sage Publications.

Mueller, F., Proctor, S. and Buchanan, D. (2000) 'Team working in its context(s): antecedents, nature and dimensions', *Human Relations*, vol 3, pp 1387-424.

NCCSDO (National Co-ordinating Centre for NHS Service Delivery and Organisation Research and Development) (2001) *Making informed decisions on change – Key points for health care managers and professionals*, London: NCCSDO.

NHSME (National Health Service Management Executive) (1993) *Nursing in primary care – New world, new opportunities*, Leeds: NHSME.

Nolan, M. (1995) 'Towards an ethos of interdisciplinary practice', *British Medical Journal*, vol 311, pp 305-7.

O'Keeffe, M., Hills, A., Doyle, M. et al (2007) *UK study of abused and neglect of older people: Prevalence survey report*, London: National Centre for Social Research.

Ojha, A.K. (2005) 'High performance organisations: discussion', *IIMB Management Review*, pp 73-91.

Onyett, S., Pillinger, T. and Muijen, M. (1997) 'Job satisfaction and burnout among members of community mental health teams', *Journal of Mental Health*, vol 6, pp 55-66.

Ouchi, W. and Johnson, A. (1978) 'Types of organisational control and their relationship to organisational well-being', *Administrative Science Quarterly*, vol 23, pp 292-317.

Øvretveit, J. (1995) 'Team decision making', *Journal of Interprofessional Care*, vol 9, pp 41-51.

Parker, R. and Bradley, L. (2000) 'Organisational culture in the public sector: evidence from six organisations', *The International Journal of Public Sector Management*, vol 13, pp 125-41.

Parker, S.K. and Williams, H.M. (2001) *Effective teamworking: Reducing the psychosocial risks*, Norwich: Health and Safety Executive.

Pasmore, W., Francis, C., Haldeman, J. and Shani, A. (1982) 'Sociotechnical systems: a North American reflection on empirical studies of the seventies', *Human Relations*, vol 35, pp 1179-204.

Payne, M. (2000) *Teamwork in multiprofessional care*, Basingstoke: Macmillan.

Pearson, P. and Jones, K. (1994) 'The primary health care non-team?', *British Medical Journal*, vol 309, pp 1387-8.

Peck, E. and Dickinson, H. (2008) *Managing and leading in inter-agency settings*, Bristol: The Policy Press.

Plsek, P. (1997) *Creativity, innovation and quality*, San Francisco, CA: ASQC Quality Press.

Poxton, R. (2004) 'What makes effective partnerships between health and social care?', in J. Glasby and E. Peck (eds) *Care trusts: Partnership working in action*, Abingdon: Radcliffe Medical Press.

Rhodes, D. (2003) *Better informed? Inspection of the management and use of information in social care*, London: Department of Health.

Richardson, S. and Asthana, S. (2005) 'Policy and legal influences on inter-organisational information sharing in health and social care services', *Journal of Integrated Care*, vol 13, pp 3-10.

Robinson, M. and Cottrell, D. (2005) 'Health professionals in multi-disciplinary and multi-agency teams: changing professional practice', *Journal of Interprofessional Care*, vol 19, pp 547-60.

Rummery, K. and Glendinning, C. (2000) *Primary care and social services: Developing new partnerships for older people*, Abingdon: Radcliffe Medical Press.

Rushmer, R. (2005) 'Blurred boundaries damage inter-professional working', *Nurse Researcher*, vol 12, pp 74-85.

Rushmer, R. and Pallis, G. (2002) 'Inter-professional working: the wisdom of integrated working and the disaster of blurred boundaries', *Public Money and Management*, pp 59-66.

Salas, E., Burke, S.C. and Cannon-Bowers, J. (2000) 'Teamwork: emerging principles', *International Journal of Management Reviews*, vol 2, pp 339-56.

Schein, E. (1985) *Organizational culture and leadership*, San Francisco, CA: Jossey-Bass.

Schultz, R. and Schultz, C. (1988) 'Management practices, physician autonomy, and satisfaction: evidence from mental health institutions in the Federal Republic of Germany', *Medical Care*, vol 26, pp 750-63.

Seddon, J. (2004) 'It's the way we work ... not the people', *Personnel Today*, 16 March.

Sheehan, D., Robertson, L. and Ormond, T. (2007) 'Comparison of language used and patterns of communication in interprofessional and multidisciplinary teams', *Journal of Interprofessional Practice*, vol 21, pp 17-30.

Sommers, L.S., Marton, K.I., Barbaccia, J.C. and Randolph, J. (2000) 'Physician, nurse and social worker collaboration in primary care for chronically ill seniors', *Archives of Internal Medicine*, vol 160, pp 1825-33.

Stanton, N. (2003) *Mastering communication*, Basingstoke: Palgrave.

Stevens, M. and Campion, M. (1994) 'The knowledge, skill, and ability requirements for teamwork: implications for human resource management', *Journal of Management*, vol 20, pp 503-30.

Sullivan, H. and Skelcher, C. (2002) *Working across boundaries: Collaboration in public services*, Basingstoke: Palgrave.

Sundstrom, E. (1999) *Supporting work team effectiveness: Best management practices for fostering high performance*, San Francisco, CA: Jossey-Bass.

- Thomas, K.W. (2002) *Introduction to conflict management: Improving performance using the TKI*, Palo Alto, CA: Consulting Psychologists Press.

Tyrer, P., Coid, J., Simmonds, S., Joseph, P. and Marriott, S. (1999) 'Community mental health teams for people with severe mental illnesses and disordered personality', *The Cochrane Library*, vol 4.

van Wijngaarden, J.D.H., de Bont, A.A. and Huijsman, R. (2006) 'Learning to cross boundaries: the integration of a health network to deliver seamless care', *Health Policy*, vol 79, pp 203-13.

Vaughan, D. (1996) *The Challenger launch decision: Risky technology, culture, and deviance at NASA*, Chicago, IL: University of Chicago Press.

Walter, J. (2005) *World disasters report 2005: Focus on information in disasters*, Geneva: International Federation of Red Cross and Red Crescent Societies.

Weick, K.E. (1987) 'Organizational culture as a source of high reliability', *California Management Review*, vol XXIX, pp 112-27.

Weldon, E. and Weingart, L. (1993) 'Group goals and group performance', *British Journal of Social Psychology*, vol 32, pp 307-34.

West, M. and Markiewicz, L. (2004) *Building team-based working: A practical guide to organizational transformation*, Leicester and Oxford: British Psychological Society and Blackwell Publishing.

West, M. and Markiewicz, L. (2006) *The effective partnership working inventory*, Working Paper, Birmingham: Aston Business School.

West, M. and Slater, J.A. (1996) *The effectiveness of team working in primary health care*, London: Health Education Authority.

West, M., Borrill, C. and Unsworth, K. (1998) 'Team effectiveness in organizations', in C.L. Cooper and I.T. Robinson (eds) *International review of industrial and organizational psychology*, vol 13, Chichester: Wiley.

Wildblood, P. (2007) 'Building effective teams' (www.management-training-consultants.com/effective-teams.htm, accessed 28/08/2007).

Young, T., Brailsford, S., Connell, C., Davies, R., Harper, P. and Klein, J.H. (2004) 'Using industrial processes to improve patient care', *British Medical Journal*, vol 328, pp 162-4.

Zwarenstein, M. and Reeves, S. (2000) 'What's so great about collaboration?: we need more evidence and less rhetoric', *British Medical Journal*, vol 7241, pp 1022-3.

Index